DISCOVERING THE
MONSTER
WITHIN

DISCOVERING THE MONSTER WITHIN

PATRICIA BURKLEY, RN
AND
JACK SUMMERS, M.D., PH.D

Pleasant Word

Pleasant Word (a division of WinePress Publishing, PO Box 428, Enumclaw, WA 98022) functions only as book publisher. As such, the ultimate design, content, editorial accuracy, and views expressed or implied in this work are those of the author.

ISBN 1-4141-0599-1
Library of Congress Catalog Card Number: 2005909036

Table of Contents

Preface

A sage once wrote, "The journey of a thousand miles begins with a single step." In my case, it began with a single bite. Although my journey is not over, I am well down the road to recovery, and like the alcoholic, I take one day at a time. My recovery is from an insidious illness that destroys not only the victims, but those around them as well.

Painted with a broad brush, I suffer from an eating disorder. The technical name for one subset of this category is Anorexia Nervosa, where victims literally starve themselves to death. In another of its diabolical categories is the subset Bulimia. Here, patients binge eat, then purge themselves with cathartics to rid the body of the loathsome food. In its worst manifestation, which afflicted me, I ate the miniscule meals of an anorexic, then purged myself like the bulimic of even those meager calories.

How I survived this deadly combination for over forty years, probably a world's record that I take no pride in, God only knows. I am convinced now that it was for a purpose. And, I believe that purpose is so I could tell my story to others in the hope that it might be a warning, a solace, or a source of inspiration.

Discovering the Monster Within

Robert Burns, the famous poet once penned:

"Oh what a gift the gods would give us,
to see ourselves as others see us."

I don't believe that I have seen myself as others see me for over four decades. Even now, when I look into the mirror, I am tempted to see the pudgy, squirrel-cheeked, obese figure instead of the rail-thin stick of a woman I had become. To tell this story, I have had to search my soul to see myself as others see me, and it has not been easy. I had to examine painful memories of abandonment, loneliness and abuse. I had to admit to my faults and how I allowed the actions of others to take away my self-respect and esteem. It was necessary to re-evaluate my marriage, my relationship with my husband and my children in the light of reality, not my perceived world.

This was a Herculean task, and could never have been accomplished on my own. God, my husband, Art, my son's, David and Calvin, and their wives, Katy and Tina, have been an integral part of my healing by giving me their unconditional love and support when they were helpless to help me, and showering me with even more love when I took charge of my life again. Also, there is my friend Monika, who was relentless with her love and relentless with her pressure to get me to take charge of my life again. To them, and the health professionals at the Remuda Ranch, and, Sarah, the lovely young woman I met there and about whom I will say more later on, I dedicate this work.

A special thanks to Sandy Derau for the dramatic art that helps capture the essence of the disease.

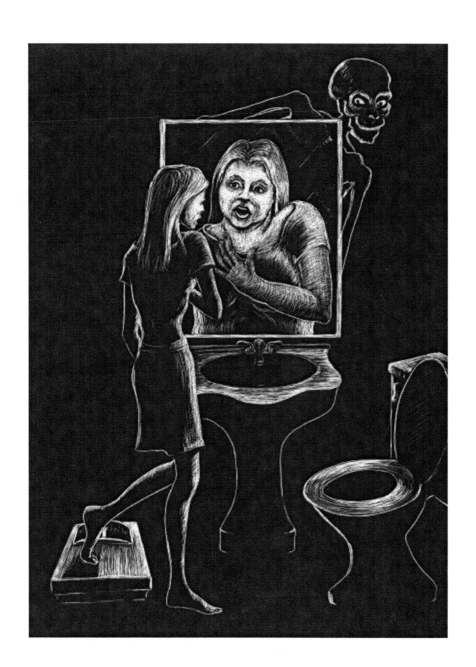

CHAPTER 1

The Beginning of the End

As my husband, Art, and I drove across the desert from our home in Las Vegas, Nevada to the insignificant town of Wickenburg, Arizona, my emotions ran the gamut from apprehension to relief as we headed into an unknown future as frightening and foreboding as an enchanted wood.

My dominant emotion was relief that I was finally going to face the monster that was slowly killing me. At the same time, I was terrified at the idea of looking deep into the core of my own being and into the monster's eyes.

The ninth chapter of the Book of Acts describes the miraculous conversion of Saul, the persecutor of Christians, to Paul, Apostle of Christ. On that dusty road in long-ago Israel, God took control of Saul's life in a direct angelic confrontation. I had no such epiphany, but the last few years of my life were marked by a gradual, grudging, argumentative negotiation with God. My angels came dressed as friends, counselors, doctors and family. He talked to me, as He usually does to stubborn, self-willed mortals, so softly that at times, I never heard Him. But, I needed your help God. Thank You for Your patience and Your persistence.

Discovering the Monster Within

At the end of the Damascus Road, Saul was led to the house of Judah, on the Street Called Straight. For three long days, he sat in the darkness, unable to see, confused and uncertain about the future. A man named Ananias was sent by the Lord to heal Saul. Placing his hands upon the grieving man's head, Ananias prayed and the scales fell away from Saul's eyes. When he arose, able to truly see for the first time in his life, he was immediately baptized and emerged from the waters of figurative death as Paul, the Apostle. Armed with his new vision, and now with an understanding of the meaning of his life, Paul carried the Christian message to the ends of the earth, never swerving from his mission that ended with his martyrdom in Rome.

Although I bear no resemblance to the disciple, our journeys are analogous. I was blind to my self destruction, stumbling through my life kicking at God's will instead of obeying it. Unable to realize that despite my efforts to do what I thought was proper, I was denying God and destroying the physical temple of my body. The scales were thick over my eyes, but also over my ears as well. Nearly every sensory input had been twisted by the bad reel on the tape player in my head and by the monster within, so that I was *totally unable* to *see or hear* the truth. And, I was dying. The house at the end of my Street Called Straight was not a house at all. Our destination was a rustic ranch in Wickenburg, Arizona called Remuda. There, my Ananias, a group of skilled healers named Rob, Julie, Dr. Gobar and a host of others would lead me through my three days of darkness.

The drive was a quiet one, each of us absorbed in our own thoughts. We knew that we were about to be separated from each other for the longest period of time in our lives, and I would be facing the biggest battle of my life without Art at my side. I knew that though he might not be physically there, he was there in spirit and each day was his battle too. It was for him as it is for so many people in wartime. Some troops are on the front line while their support staff sits miles away hanging on every piece of news from the front lines. And, we both knew that this was a desperate battle that I must win.

12

The Beginning of the End

There was one consolation as the monotonous miles droned by. I finally knew, beyond all doubt, that God loved me, and He was with me, too. I could feel God's love as tangibly as I could Art's. That love, and my will to live drove with me toward our destination.

Looking across the seat at the man I love, I became painfully aware of another truth. Art had been a good and patient husband, sharing me with my monster for over four decades. Much of Art's personal pain came from the monster's possession of me. He deserved more than the sickly, self-destructive, weak, self-centered shrew I had become. Just as importantly, I didn't deserve to be such a vial creature. After all, God, and Art Burkley loved me, and that made me important. That was the truth, and that truth would set me free.

I made my decision. I had to do this or die. For forty years I'd been tying to ignore the monster inside of me. The monster is as hideous as any medieval gargoyle and as deadly as cancer. Its invasion was insidious, spawned by a simple act of rebellion and ending with total control of my life and my body. The demon's name is anorexia, and I must exorcise it or die.

The unimposing white Rancho Remuda, with a distinctive, red-tiled roof looked more like the residence of a prosperous Spanish Don than it did the battleground where combat with monsters raged. Accent landscape lights outlined the trim walkway, and Saguaro Cactus stood on each side of the path reminding my overworked imagination of oriental temple guardians.

Reaching for the doorknob of the Remuda Ranch Treatment Center for Anorexic Women, every fiber of my being screamed for me to run! Turn around and dash down the path; leap into the car; slam the door and snap down the door locks! Was it really my *emotions* that were begging me to flee, or was it my *eating disorder*, that I have personified as ED, yammering in my head? Of course, ED is a *he,* since the dominant players in each act of my life have been men. Wrapping my skeletal fingers around the knob, I ignored the strident voice of ED and stepped inside.

Discovering the Monster Within

Art and I approached the registration area with all the confidence of Hansel and Gretel in the witch's kitchen. When we reached the desk, what little bravado I had left wavered. Anyone who even gave me a casual glance could see that I was fighting a loosing battle with starvation. ED was so strong. How could I ever hope to beat him? I was alone, vulnerable.

As I signed in, and filled out the prerequisite registration forms, I came face-to-face with one of the first realities of living with ED. It's cheap to get into it, and expensive to get out of it. When your daily diet matches that of a psychotic rabbit, you don't spend much on groceries. Lettuce is cheap. But, reputable treatment programs will cost as much as $30,000 for outpatient therapies to over $100,000 for inpatient ones. Remuda was a bargain at only $70,000 for sixty days of in-patient therapy. With a sigh of resignation, I left admitting and entered the patients living quarters.

Walking down the hall, my heart was in my throat. Unsure of what to expect, I was shocked and dismayed by what I saw. Wide, haunted eyes tinged with fear stared curiously at me from black circled sockets. When I looked directly at one person, she avoided eye contact with me and bowed her head with what . . . shame? Like ancient gnomes in a forgotten dungeon, skeletal bodies were everywhere. Was I one of them? No! I was *fat*, not one of these starving creatures! That's what ED told me, and I believed him.

One difference between the others and me was immediately striking. I was old enough to be the mother of all of them, and in a few cases, the grandmother of some of them. Were they wondering what I was doing here? My hands began to shake as shame scalded my cheeks, and I was consumed by the profound sorrow that I had waited this long to reach out for help. It was going to be hard for me to face them, but I had to. With a tilt of my chin, I steeled my resolve. I'm tired of being a victim! I want my life back!

As a nurse, I learned a great deal about nutrition. Realizing I had a problem, I learned a lot about anorexia. I learned the facts intellectually, as one might know how a clock works from reading an article about the subject. I *knew* the facts, but they had *no substance* for me. I knew exactly how many calories per day a healthy five feet seven inches tall woman like me needed to maintain an ideal weight. Then, how did I become the scarecrow I was when I checked into the Ranch? The answer is simple, although rational people find it nearly impossible to understand. At that point in my life, I would rather have died than gain an ounce! I prayed to God that at Remuda I might find out why I felt that way.

Although those of us who harbor the monster are living testimony to the ability of the human body to survive on starvation rations for extended periods of time, Anorexia is *not* about food. Anorexia is a symptom of a complex disease involving control issues, self-esteem, perfectionism, mood swings, shame, guilt, depression and all-or-none thinking. And, those were just the emotional and behavioral things involved. There are physical ones, too.

Getting into the treatment center at Remuda wasn't easy. First, I had to qualify. Being female was a good start, since more than ninety percent of us with ED are women. That's not a statistic that women's organizations tend to tout.

Next, I needed to be fifteen percent below my normal body weight for age and height. Since I had been a practicing anorexic for forty-two consecutive years, I qualified on this one at every age for the last forty years. In fact, many therapists have told me that I may be one of the longest continuous practitioners of anorexia known. Most people with the disease have either short periods of self-abuse, or will take a few years off and eat normally before falling back into the clutches of the disease. Or, the disease kills them, as it did Karen Carpenter, the popular singer. I don't plan to include more than forty years of self starvation in my resume.

I also had to miss three consecutive periods. Been there; done that. Thirty-years ago I missed three periods. After my third child was born, periods stopped altogether, except for inconsistent cramping and spotting that lead to an eventual hysterectomy. I passed that test without cramming.

The next hurdles were more ephemeral, but certainly not obstacles. One was body image. My view of my body was as distorted as if I had been looking into a fun-house mirror. When I looked at my reflection, I saw an obese, bloated, acne-scarred woman, who needed to lose weight desperately, instead of the eighty-two pound scarecrow I really was.

My final challenge was that I needed to be deathly afraid of gaining weight. No, problem again. Since I had been existing, I won't call it living, on four hundred calories a day or less, my actions spoke for themselves.

At least I was in good company. In his entertaining book with the catchy title of *Holy Anorexia*, Rudolph M. Bell reported some interesting reasons for anorexia. He relates the strange life of Catherine Benincassa, or Saint Catherine of Sienna , who lived in 1373, and was a severe anorexic. She staunchly defended her self-destructive action as direct orders from God. Saint Clair of Assisi, companion of Saint Francis who lived in 1253, was also a fellow traveler. According to Bell, nearly half of the forty-two thirteenth Century women who later became saints exhibited anorexic behavior at some time in their life. I certainly never claimed that God, or the Devil, made me do it. I just knew I would never get out of it without God's help.

Then, it came time to say good-by to my darling husband. He was heading back home, and I was concerned because he was making the long drive alone. When he walked out that door, I felt my heart and my security go with him.

I knew that he got home okay, because he left me a message to that effect. For the first seventy-two hours, we were not allowed to communicate with anyone on the outside. When he was still working and traveling for B. F. Goodrich, he called me nearly every night to touch base, fill me in on his day and see how mine went. This would be the longest we had ever gone without talking to each other. Ordinarily, I don't worry about Art traveling, but I needed something else to worry about so I wouldn't think about what I had to start doing tomorrow. I thanked God that the trip was uneventful. Focusing on God, as I did every spare moment while I was there, I slept more soundly than I could have dreamed possible.

The first order of business at the Ranch was a complete history and physical examination as well as a full laboratory evaluation and EKG. A prior trip to the Mayo Clinic in Scottsdale, Arizona had diagnosed severe osteoporosis. The Remuda doctors were as appalled as the Scottsdale crew by my serum calcium levels.

The only time I was allowed to violate the rules at Remuda was due to the severity of my osteoporosis, common baggage for many anorexics. I was a sleepwalker, and once, when I was put on a new medication, the folks at the ranch were afraid I might trip and fall, so I was allowed to sleep on a cot in the living room instead of my bedroom. Though, I didn't take one of my zombie strolls for them, it was a wise decision.

Because of the osteoporosis, I was not fully able to participate in the ranch's equine therapy program. Every resident, they never called us patients, is assigned a horse while at the ranch. Many of us had never seen a horse outside a Saturday matinee, but we were assigned to feed, groom, care for and ride a lovely animal. The lesson is to teach us that if we can control a thousand pounds of horseflesh, we can control our own lives. I was able to bond with my horse, and I lead her around and groomed her every day, but I never rode. They were afraid that if I fell off, I would shatter like a china doll.

Next was the nutritional assessment. At my weigh in, I tipped the scales at a whopping eighty-two pounds. A plan to restore my weight using caloric intake based ideal body weight and percent of body fat, of which I possessed none, was calculated. Muttering to themselves, my new inquisitors trotted off to devise a diabolical torture, called a menu, using the weapon I feared the most in life . . . food.

We quickly established a routine that was scary, strange, humbling and down right hard! In some ways, they treated us like prisoners on a cell block. Hair driers, along with glass perfume bottles, or any item the staff considered dangerous, were kept at the nurses station and had to be signed in and out! We had a number of rules about everything from what we wore to what we ate.

I considered the first few days of therapy miner's week. It was spent in interviews, written tests and more interviews. They were digging into me as a coal miner attacks a coal seam, to see what psychological and emotional damage had been done to me to produce the ravaged body that I brought with me to the Ranch. It was considerable. At week's end, I met my Ananias fill-ins, my counselor, Rob, nutritionist, Julie, and psychiatrist, Dr. Gobar, a sociologist and a member of the medical staff. That night, I didn't sleep as well. The opening salvo of my war with ED would be fired in the morning.

"Please, God," I prayed as I pulled up the sheet. "Give me the strength I need."

CHAPTER 2

Home Sweet Pain

Therapy at Remuda is nutritional, spiritual, experiential and psychiatric. Counseling of every ilk is included. It includes individual psychotherapy, group therapy, and subspecialty groups for those with addictions, victims of sexual abuse, obsessive compulsive behavior and any other problem that could be imagined. Rob was my primary psychologist, and with his skilled guidance, we peeled the stages of my life like an onion, removing one facade after another to expose the diseased layer beneath.

Anorexia nervosa is a Latin term whose literal meaning is "nervous want of appetite." And, it is a killer. According to published statistics, even in its mildest manifestation, one person in ten dies. But, I doubt the validity of those figures. I believe that thousands of us go undiagnosed and die from our disease while more fashionable diagnoses take credit for the kill. I believe that because with the countless visits I had over the years with physicians, therapists, psychologists and councilors, *no one ever* addressed my real disease. The dentist fixed my teeth that I was scalding to withered stumps with the hydrochloric stomach acid from my purging, but never broached the cause. Physicians treated my broken bones, prescribed for my nutritionally related ailments but never confronted me about my behavior. As a group, anorexics are ignored.

A more discouraging figure relates to relapse rates. Only half of us who successfully complete therapy remain in remission at two years. I am determined to be in the permanently cured half.

Conservatively, seven million women in the United States are identified as anorexic. Despite the fact that eating disorders are rampant, very few states have programs to combat either anorexia or bulimia. A miniscule number of colleges have programs to educate the youth of America about the dangers of eating disorders. That figure is tragic, since over eighty percent of women with anorexia have symptoms by age twenty, which included yours truly.

The disease is indeed a "nervous want of appetite," with an emphasis on the nervous part. Low self esteem was but one of a host of "nervous" components that made it possible for ED to germinate and bloom in me. A great deal of one's self esteem is established early in life by interaction with the nuclear family, and mine was damaged as early in my life as my memory allows me to remember.

I came into this world, May 27th, 1940 in Johnson City, New York, the third child of Lucille Pearl Schilpp and Calvin Reynolds Archer. My eldest sister, Beverly, was five, and my other sister, Linda, was eighteen months when the event, which my parents did not treat as blessed, transpired.

I have no record of the weather on the spring day I was born. It may have been bright and sunny or tossed with the thunderstorms so common to spring in New York. From the Archer family's point of view, my birth was as welcome as Pearl Harbor would be to the country nineteen months later.

Unwanted, and unplanned, I was the product of a difficult labor, which my parents made plain to me as soon as I was old enough to understand. There was never enough money to go around, and the two girls they already had were enough. In addition, I was a large baby, with broad shoulders, and my mother was devastated when the doctor told her she would never have her boy because of the damage done to her reproductive organs by my pregnancy. Good old Pat was down two strikes to the pitcher of life, and I wasn't even out of the delivery room yet.

Had I been a boy, these prenatal sins might have been forgiven. Instead, I was simply another burden to be endured, another mouth to be fed. Because of my parent's desperate desire for a son, and most devastating of all to me, I was invariably introduced as "Patricia, who should have been Patrick, but we love her anyway." I was never sure whether that meant that they loved me or not. As a child, it confirmed to me that my place in this family was on shaky ground.

If my evaluation of the situation sounds harsh, it shouldn't. I'm not alone in these circumstances. I know a woman who was named Tommy, because she was the sixth girl in a family that desired a son with every fiber of their being. When her mother discovered she had delivered another daughter, she said to the shocked obstetrician, "Take it back. I don't want another girl." Now in the twilight of her life, when Tommy relates those cruel words, the tone of her voice still carries traces of the pain it has caused her. All her life, Tommy felt the same uncertainties about her nuclear family as I did mine.

The obstetrician told Tommy's mother to keep the baby for few days, and if she decided then she didn't want her, he would take her back. Of course her mother kept her, but later in life, each time she displeased her mother, she was chastised with, "I should have given you back." Even as an adult, Tommy was never certain how serious her mother was when she said it. "This is Patricia. She should have been Patrick, but we love her anyway," cut me the same way. Tommy has an eating disorder, but it's the opposite of mine. All her life she has been overweight.

My formative years are a series of memories, some as vivid as yesterday while others are shrouded in the haze of half a century, but all indelibly tied to three houses in Ohio. They were the houses on Sycamore Street, Midway and Johnny Cake. It is difficult for me to call them homes, for each of them was a house of pain for me. Despite the fact that they were houses where my family lived, and each had its share of memories that are precious to me, they were still merely places where I existed until I could escape. They are a perfect example of the many ambivalences of my childhood. All these houses are in Lake County, Ohio near the city of Painesville.

The town's name is apropos because pain is among my earliest recollections from the house on Sycamore Street where we lived until I was seven. In many houses of that period, the heat was transmitted through ducts covered by metal grates that came up through the floor. Those grates became a painful part of my childhood, as they did for countless other toddlers back then. At age four, lurching about the house, I stumbled and landed with both palms on the grate.

Pain from those burns remains etched in my brain as one of my earliest memories of my childhood. My mother did her best to sooth them. She covered my hands with salve and bandages cut from an old sheet. She had nothing to give me for the pain. Fortunately, there was no permanent damage or scarring.

Parents send children all sorts of confusing and subliminal messages, and the translation of those messages by the child is often a galaxy's distance from what the parent intended. For example, "That's not the way to do it. Let me show you how," can be translated by the child as, "I'm such a klutz. I can't do anything right." "Why is your face always dirty?" comes out, "I'm a dirty person." And, as was my case, "Don't wear that skirt. It's too tight." Ignoring a recent growth spurt, my read was, "I'm too fat."

When the pattern is repeated too often, as it was in my case, I arrived at the conclusion that, "I'm not who I thought I was. I thought I was okay, but it seems I'm a fat, worthless, slob who can't do anything right. "

I heard that song so many times as a child, I decided to join the choir. I did, and at sixty years of age, like most other anorexics, I didn't have a clue as to who the real me was.

Since my parents played a major role in sending me these messages, I should introduce them. My mother was five feet-four inches tall with blond hair and an angular build. She was an attractive woman, whose weight fluctuated between one hundred-thirty and one hundred-fifty pounds, depending upon her stress levels and state of her health at the moment. Looking into the mirror, I heard her say a hundred times, "If my butt gets any bigger, I'm not gonna fit on the couch." It was an early lesson for this little girl. Broad butts are not good!

Those early years of my life were filled with chaos and open warfare between my parents, but Mom remained even-tempered with us children. By every yardstick, then or now, we would have been considered poor, so she spent a great deal of her time trying to compensate for what we didn't have; to make holidays special for us and to be the stable counterpoint to my father's instability. Despite her role as peacemaker, Mom was a strong, stubborn personality in her own right, and this trait contributed to much of the tension in the Archer household. Without her love and devotion to us during this time, I shudder to think of what might have happened to me.

Even as a child, I felt a strange mixture of fear and alienation as I began, even then, to slip into the victim's role. I felt as if I was alone; the outsider, who wasn't wanted. I could never permanently rid myself of those feelings no matter how much I tried.

Calvin Archer was an inch shy of six feet tall and never weighed more than one hundred-fifty pounds. A straight, prominent nose dominated a long, dark face surrounded by equally dark hair that thinned early. A handsome man, he was nicknamed, "Lindy," for his resemblance to the famous aviator, Charles Lindbergh.

My father had a short and difficult life. When I was born, he was alone in the world, except for our family. His mother and father both died young, and by the time he was ten, he was living with relatives and in foster homes. Forced by circumstance and the Great Depression, he began working then, too. I have often wondered if his profound lack of family and the nurturing that is so key to a healthy adult might have been the cause for some of my father's problems. At the very least, he was robbed of his childhood, as were many caught in the economic catastrophe of those terrible times.

He was a construction worker when we moved to Ohio, and one of the first projects he worked on was the Fulton Road Bridge at the Cleveland Zoo. It remained a constant reminder of him while we lived in the area. Later, he worked for Diamond Alkali in Painesville, Ohio. Volatile and quick-tempered, his personality best resembled a ticking bomb, and we never knew when it would go off. He never slapped us or beat us, and any sort of corporal punishment was rare, but he could skin you alive with words.

At best, the relationship between my parents could be characterized as stormy. They were two strong personalities, which lead to frequent and divisive confrontations. Mom kept her father, Grandpa Wally Schilpp, on a pedestal. No matter how hard he tried, my father could never measure up to the legendary proportions mother assigned to Grandfather. Any small incident was enough to start a new war. Unfortunately, my father provided her with an ample supply of ammunition for her verbal Gattling gun.

Some of my earliest memories of my father were of him stumbling around the house so drunk he could barely maneuver. One warm, summer night, when I was around five, I was sound asleep when my mother entered our bedroom. Obviously distressed, her face was flushed and stained with tears.

"Get up, girls. I need your help right now!" she said with a desperation that prompted immediate compliance.

"Mommy, what's wrong?" Beverly asked, uncertainty tingeing my big sister's voice and raising my anxiety titer higher than it already was.

"Get up and get out to the car *now!*" my mother shouted, her voice pitch approaching hysteria. Turning she hurried from the bedroom.

Tugging on clothes, we ran barefoot outside. Shoes were not part of our summer attire. They were too expensive. What was wrong? I couldn't understand what was happening. I started to cry without understanding why.

Home Sweet Pain

The driver's door to the family car was open, and Mom was waiting with a blanket and bucket of water. I could see my father slumped over the steering wheel.

Something bad has happened to him! He's dead! He must be dead!" I thought. Although I had only a five year old's perspective of death, I knew it was not a good thing. Tears ran down my cheeks, and I began to sob.

When I got closer, my stomach churned at the awful stench emanating from inside the car. My head swam, and I leaned against the car as I wretched. He wasn't dead. He had thrown up and passed out . . . drunk again, as mom was so fond of reiterating.

"Help me get him out of the car, now!" mom wailed.

Straining, we complied and with great difficulty wrestled him from behind the steering wheel onto the grass. Trying to support the dead weight of one leg, I slipped and fell on my butt. Besides the vomit, he had soiled himself, too. Gagging, I sat in the mire and cried until my sisters spurred me back into action.

I have no idea how long it took to drag him to the outhouse, but it seemed like an eternity. Wrangling him inside like a hog-tied calf, we propped him against the privy wall.

"Get those filthy clothes off him and clean him up," Mom commanded.

"Yuck! I can't do that. He's all slimy!" Beverly complained.

"Yeah, Yuck!" I agreed, praying with a child's naiveté that I would be sent back to bed.

"Now damn it! Get busy!" Mom snarled.

Working like demented gnomes, we stripped him down to his shorts and scrubbed his face, hands and neck while he blubbered unintelligibly. By the time we finished, and trundled him off to bed, the night was nearly gone. Going to the wash basin, like a pint-sized Lady Macbeth, I washed my hands over and over. I scrubbed them until I was afraid the skin would come off, but they still didn't feel clean. I cleaned the rest of my little body as much as the washbasin would allow.

Discovering the Monster Within

Crawling into bed, I stared at the ceiling afraid to go to sleep because I was unreasonably convinced that something bad would happen to my father if I drifted off. I lay there tossing and turning until fatigue eventually overwhelmed me. My red rimmed eyes burned, and I remember wondering how much a person could cry. It seemed as if the tears would never stop. When sleep finally claimed me, it was with dread of the next morning.

At Remuda, we learned a great deal about conflict resolution. Too often, conflicts are settled in a straight forward win/lose format. The winner fulfills their need at the expense of the loser. Compromise is a better option that can be a win-win solution for both parties in the end. Alas that was not in my parent's armamentarium.

Compromise requires that both parties shift the focus from themselves to the other person, or the relation they have with the other combatant. That was out of the question for my father, whose entire world revolved around himself, and for my mother whose will of iron did not include losing. The only conflict resolution I ever saw was the lose/lose technique, vividly illustrated by the battling Archers the next morning.

Shouts from the kitchen awakened me, and I burrowed into the pillow, covering my ears to blot out the noise. It didn't work.

"I don't care," my mother shouted. "There was lipstick all over your shirt. You were with that bitch again, weren't you? I've had about all of this I can take, you bastard!"

Her angry expletive was punctuated by the sound of breaking pottery.

"God damn you! I'm going to smack the shit out of you!" my father roared to the accompaniment of an overturning chair.

The fear I felt was like a living thing trying to suffocate me. I wanted to scream for them to stop, but I couldn't get enough air into my lungs to make a sound. My sisters stared at me wide-eyed. None of us had a clue as to what we should do, so we cowered.

"Touch me and I'm calling the cops!" Mom yells back.

Home Sweet Pain

Another crash reverberates from the kitchen.

"I can't stand you! I can't stand this place. You . . . those damned brats!"

Moments later, the front door slammed and an ominous silence settled over the house. In time, the quiet was disturbed by heart-rending sobs from the kitchen.

Although my father was never physically abusive with us, he was with my mother. And, she gave as well as received. I remember another infamous brawl. Although I'm not exactly sure what started it, it had to be drinking, money, gambling or women. All the others were.

As my sisters and I sat frozen in terror, we could hear them screaming at each other. Slaps, grunts, punches and crashing furniture summoned a new flood of tears from the three of us. A loud clunk, followed by a louder than usual bellow of rage, drove me to the door despite knees that threatened to buckle with fear. My father was headed toward his bedroom, blood streaming down his face from a gash over his left eye. In the doorway to the kitchen, Mom stood triumphantly with a frying pan in her hand, her split upper lip beginning to swell grotesquely.

When things got this out of hand, we were frequently spirited away to the Stephens' house across the street. I don't remember much about them, except that they were kind, compassionate people whose home became a sanctuary to us.

Today, the Archer house would be a regular stop on police rounds, and Children's Services Board caseworkers would have been on a first name basis. Fifty years ago, spouses duked it out, and children were caught in the crossfire. My sisters and I had a ringside seat.

For days after each bout, I tiptoed around the house, trying not to be more of a problem than I had already been told I was. By now, I was firmly convinced that I was the major reason for my parent's routine battles. Look at the trouble I caused by just being born.

Remuda teaches that communication is on two levels, the superficial, where facts and information are exchanged, and the intimate, where feelings and self are explored. All humans need both kinds, but talking about feelings is scary. There is too much chance the person to whom you are baring your soul will say, "I don't care." Equally appalling, they might take your words and turn them against you. Since my parents couldn't ever communicate in that fashion, they used their daughters in a classic, dysfunctional, communication triangle instead.

After some of their championship level fights, like the one just described, first my mother, then my father would isolate each of us. I'll never forget those conversations.

Setting me on the edge of the bed, Mom would pull a chair up in front of me.

"Pat, honey, you know Daddy and Mommy don't get along. You hear us fighting and arguing. We are probably going to get a divorce. Do you know what a divorce is?"

I shook my head no the first time we had this conversation.

"A divorce means that Daddy and Mommy will not be living together any more. You kids will have to decide whether you live with your dad or me. Do you understand?"

Tears streaming down my face, trembling with emotion, I nodded my head. I really didn't understand, but I knew it was what she wanted me to do. I was learning to please at an early age, even if the action caused me untenable levels of anxiety.

"When the lawyers ask you, you tell them you want to live with me, Sweetie. Okay?"

Unable to speak, I could only nod.

Later that day, I had the same conversation with my father, agreeing to live with him, too. I didn't know what else to do. What would happen if I ever *really* had to decide between them? What would I do? The possibility of having to make that decision overwhelmed me, and it drove me to the edge of a mental breakdown.

From that horrific experience, I learned a primitive survival skill that would prove invaluable to me in years to come. I found I could disassociate my feelings from reality and save myself from the final leap to madness. Ruthlessly repressing my emotions, I drove them deep inside myself. I literally forced myself not to think about them except in an abstract way. It was as if it was happening to someone else, and I was only a bystander. It allowed my five-year-old mind to survive intact, but plowed the field where the monster would be planted.

Unfortunately, these conversations were repeated more than once. Fortunately, the majority of them were seldom face-to-face. Usually, they called us at the Stephens' home and talked to each of us on the phone. That made it only slightly less traumatic. I don't understand how the Stephens' family was able to tolerate these episodes, but thank God they did.

Throughout the ordeal, I was faced with a problem insoluble to my childhood ability to reason. If I was such a terrible child, one they wished had never been born, and caused their problems in the first place, why did either of them want me to go with them? Why would they care? Why wouldn't my dad try to get me to go with my mother, or vice versa?

This left me with an ominous sense of foreboding. What if my *parents* came to that conclusion, too? They could both leave me. In the dead of night, they might steal away leaving me *alone!* Every day, I lived in fear, afraid that some innocuous action would be the last straw for the camel's back, and they would leave me forever. If they left, I knew they would take my sisters and leave me. They really didn't want me. I wasn't Patrick. Relying on my new skill of disassociation, I internalized my fears where they festered.

Despite my parents' volatile lifestyle, they did have friends. Unfortunately, they were as dysfunctional as my parents. Perhaps likes do attract. As role models, they were sorely lacking.

Marjorie and Sonny lived nearby. They were the only friends that seemed close to my mother. Sonny, a victim of childhood polio, was a tyrant. Using his disability like a whip, he was dominating, cruel and selfish.

Discovering the Monster Within

The opposite of her mate, Marjorie was a compliant draft horse who tirelessly pulled the load of the whole family. She spent every waking moment waiting on Sonny hand and foot.

"Get me a glass of water. Bring me dinner. Turn down the heat," were Sonny's kinder words to his devoted wife.

I remember her as a wonderful person. A treat for the Archer sisters was a chance to spend the night with Marjorie. But, she would only take us one at a time, because three of us at once were too much trouble. I was positive that the real reason we couldn't all go together was me. I was so much trouble; she couldn't handle my sisters *and me*. And, she was too nice to take the two of them without me. When Marjorie died prematurely, my mother blamed Sonny for stealing Marjorie's life from her. Mom never forgave him.

Their other friends were Eva and Donald. Donald's disability was self-inflicted. He was morbidly obese from the constant consumption of food. Alice, the cheerful enabler, cooked and served him enormous piles of anything edible. This time, it was the husband's turn for an early death as Donald succumbed to cardiac arrest in his early fifties.

From these exemplary role models, I learned two things. If you were obedient enough, and subjugated yourself enough, even a son-of-a-bitch, like Sonny, could be appeased. Second, I vowed that I would never, never, never be a fat, greasy slob like Donald. If I stayed thin, I might escape the early death he inflicted upon himself. My first eating disorder lesson learned, the monster's initial incursion into my body was so painless I never felt it.

Marjorie and Sonny provide me with one of the more pleasant memories of my time on Sycamore Street. They decided to build a grocery store, and my parents helped them dig the foundation. It took quite some time to complete the project, since they could only dig evenings after work and on weekends. Of course, Sonny couldn't dig at all.

Our parents' labor turned into a dazzling opportunity for the Archer girls to exercise the imaginations they spawned during the hours spent playing on the foundation. The piles of dirt became the mountains the settlers had to cross to reach the Promised Land. Indians lurked behind every one, but our imaginary men-folk, who were always kind, loving and polite, protected us.

Other times, they were sand dunes, inhabited by hostile Bedouins. If it were not for the brave Foreign Legionnaires, who were always kind, loving and polite, we would have been enslaved in a harem. My older sisters supplied the plots, but my fertile imagination filled in the blanks, even if I didn't know what a harem was. I just knew it was a place I didn't want to go.

The dirt piles were mountaintops from which I could look down on the whole world. Best of all, Oz lay at the end of the yellow brick road that wound its way among the dirt piles. Toto and I skipped down that road and made it to Oz despite the efforts of the Wicked Witch. The joys of that summer nearly matched the pain of it.

My father used any holiday, and particularly Christmas, as an excuse for more prodigious consumption. As my sisters and I sorted noisily through the meager tree decorations, our father attempted to place a live tree into a three pronged tree stand. The tree was too large, and the trunk bent at a slight angle. When he got the tree into the holder at the proper attitude to make it reasonably straight, the weight of the tree was too much for the inexpensive stand, and the tree toppled over. With a string of his usual colorful metaphors, he flew into one of his sudden rages. Storming to the kitchen, he returned with a hammer and nails and nailed the Christmas tree stand to the floor.

We fled to the bedroom, quaking in shock and dismay. Afraid to come out, we huddled there like homeless urchins until he had gone back to the kitchen to refill his empty glass, and Mom began to decorate the tree.

As an adult I realize that my father's hair trigger, fogged by too much cheap whiskey, catalyzed the outburst. On *that* day, I was positive it was something else. It was triggered by something I did, or said. I would have to be extra careful as I began the New Year, or I might be nailed to the floor for being such a terrible child. The victim's mentality that would blight the rest of my life was properly ingrained.

Near the end of our Sycamore Street sojourn, the baby that I should have been was born, despite the so-called irreversible damage I had done to the reproduction facility with my line backer's shoulders. April first, nineteen forty-six, David Byron Archer, (my father named him after his friend Sonny), became the fourth child in the family. My father found it impossible to believe that he had his boy. His conversation with the obstetrician has become a family legend.

The obstetrician came into the waiting room to find my father smoking, pacing and likely pining for his next drink.

"Mr. Archer, you have a bouncing baby boy!" the doctor exclaimed.

"Yeah, right, just show me which girl is mine," Calvin said dejectedly.

"No, it's not a girl. It's a boy," the doctor replied.

"Look, Doc, cut the bullshit. Do you think I'm stupid? We both know its April Fool's Day. Just show her to me so I can get the hell out of here!"

"Really, Mr. Archer, it *is a boy*!" the irritated doctor shot back.

"Damn it doc! I said that's enough bullshit! If it's a boy, prove it to me!"

Stomping back to the nursery, the doctor returned with my brother in a blanket. Throwing open the garment to show my father the prerequisite equipment to connote a male, he said, "Now, have you ever seen a girl with one of these?"

My flabbergasted father could only shake his head in disbelief. Of course, that was a real reason for my father to celebrate . . . and he did.

I celebrated, too. They now had proof that my birth did not damage my mom's anatomy badly enough to prevent the birth of the son they so desperately wanted. Had they known that all along and just used it against me because they didn't want me? My six-year-old brain couldn't sort out so weighty a question.

Beverly, now twelve, and Linda, a little over seven, were excited about the possibility of having a real baby brother to play with and take care of. I had a different spin on the grand event. In my child's heart lurked the dread that now that they had their son, this boy I should have been, how long would it be before he would take my place in the family? My parents always argued over money and were constantly telling us there was not enough for the five of us. Now there were six. Would they stop feeding me, kick me out in the street or send me away to live with some stranger? If they did, where would I go? What would I do? These thoughts caused me untold hours of anxiety and sleeplessness.

Dave did prove to be a source of joy and entertainment. He was our wonder kid. Led by Beverly, we dressed him up, took him for rides in his buggy and generally doted over him. When he got the chicken pox, we helped give him an oatmeal bath in his bath-a-net. In time, I resented the intruder less as I came to a realization that, at least for the time being, he wasn't going to get me kicked out of the house.

An indelible incident linked to Dave's childhood occurred just before we left Sycamore Street. The three of us had been left in the car to mind Dave while my parents went into a friend's house for a moment. It was a warm day, and the car windows were open. As we squabbled over something inconsequential, Dave crawled through the window and fell onto the gravel driveway lacerating his eyebrow.

When my parents responded to the screaming children, my mother began to cry and try to sooth Dave in a fashion that bordered on panic. My father reacted accordingly and flew into a rage filled with cursing and incrimination. A frantic ride to the emergency room followed where David's laceration was sutured.

When we got home, both parents attacked us verbally, my father wielding his acid tongued vocabulary with the skill of a muleskinner's whip. Beverly, being the eldest, received the brunt of the lashes, but Linda and I knew we were equally to blame.

Discovering the Monster Within

The years on Sycamore Street thus hold a bittersweet combination of good times and bad. I have many treasured memories as well as nightmares. During that time, I felt more fear, pain, anger and separation anxiety than any child should have to endure. Yet mixed with it all was a burning desire to prove to my father and mother that it was okay for me to be part of the family. That was made doubly difficult because I had yet to develop any sense of self-worth. I could not think of a single reason why they would want me to be part of their family. I had no individuality. I spent all my time trying to blend in and stay unnoticed. I wanted my family to accept me, take me in, nourish me, protect me, and allow me to be a loved part of it. This dysfunctional family unit was like a mindless robot that fed on my pain and was bent on my destruction.

Both of my parents changed by the time we moved to our third house on Johnny Cake, and in neither one was it for the better. My father became what modern psychologists call a Dry Drunk. He stopped drinking and joined Alcoholic's Anonymous, but the negative aspects of his personality remained and magnified. Although he became less physically violent, his razor sharp tongue became more damaging than any punch could ever be.

Already an expert on most things, he became an expert on everything. He hated everyone with a formal education that exceeded his grammar school equivalent. Anyone who had a high school education was a simpleton lacking the common sense of a goose. If the person by chance possessed a college degree, he was a worthless prick. My father was a male chauvinist pig of the first order. If you were female, your only value was as a breeder. Independent thought was discouraged, opinions contrary to his not tolerated and disagreement with a male, particularly him, was a mortal sin for which there was no atonement.

No one escaped his verbal fury. His interactions with my mother were cutting, sarcastic and cruel. Their verbal exchanges were more frequent and far more brutal than their physical battles ever were. Since they seldom spoke a civil word to each other, it set the tone for constant tension.

My sisters and I could never please him. He constantly harped on us for leaving a light on, standing at the refrigerator with the door open, or playing the radio too loud. We were afraid to do almost anything lest his wrath fall on us like an avalanche.

I remember a particular occasion when I needed to press a dress for school the next day. As I was setting up the ironing board and plugging in the iron, he came into the room.

"What the hell do you think you're doing?" he snarled.

"I have to press my dress for school," I answered, fear creeping into me as it always did when he lashed me with his words.

"What else are you ironing?" he demanded with a snarl.

"Just the dress. It won't take long. I'll put everything away when I'm done," I said.

Walking to the outlet, he yanked the plug from the socket.

"Put that God damned thing away. You're not gonna waste electricity heating an iron for one dress. You stupid little shit!"

Turning, he strode angrily from the room as I fumbled to put the ironing board away.

Living amidst so much turmoil, it was easy for my unsophisticated childhood logic to mold my personality into one of self-loathing, although I didn't call it that then. I only knew that I felt that my parents really didn't want me. I was nothing but trouble for them, and I felt I would never fit into the family. If I stayed quiet, tried not to cause too much trouble, them maybe, just maybe, they'd let me stay in the family.

CHAPTER 3

Pull the Trigger

All anorexics and bulimics feel that their lives are out of control. The disease is about getting control of the life which the anorexic views as not only out of control but worthless. The only thing I felt I was truly able to control was what I ate, or didn't eat. During therapy, a careful search is made for something that triggered the behavior.

When the trigger is pulled, a point, or locus, of control is disrupted. If that locus can be identified, and is not severe, the eating disorder may be easier to treat. If it is multifaceted, as was mine, treatment becomes more complex. The younger the person is when control is lost, the more difficult it is to identify and the more ingrained the inappropriate coping mechanism becomes. Once the locus of control is disrupted, the perception of a life careening out of control is the result, and something must be done to right the ship.

The onset of puberty is a common trigger. As the female body begins to develop, it loses its little girl look forever ending the illusion of perpetual youth. Some of us cannot accept this natural event, and try to starve ourselves back into pre-pubescent childhood. Child star Tracy Gold, in her biography, *Room To Grow; An Appetite for Life*, illustrates this

36

characteristic in graphic detail. As her body began to grow and develop, she tried to cling to the little girl look that had been the keystone of her acting career. Although puberty played a roll in my problem, it was merely the second trigger on the double barreled shotgun of tragedies that set me on the inevitable road to disaster.

One of the first body image events and the difference between boys and girls that I can remember was when I turned eight. On my eighth birthday, Mom took us on an outing to the Cleveland Art Museum. It was a wonderland of beautiful things. My sisters and I were particularly enamored with the nude statues, which we though were a hoot.

Looking at a marble statue of an ancient Roman soldier, we all noticed his lance, and not the one in his hand. "Look it! Look it!" Beverly exclaimed. Being the oldest, and the most knowledgeable of worldly things, she was always our leader into mischief.

Giggling her high pitched giggle, Linda covered her mouth in a partially successful attempt to stifle a shriek. I stared, open-mouthed and transfixed for a moment before joining in the reverie.

The rest of the morning, we gawked, pointed and tittered to the utter dismay of Mom, who tried valiantly to avert our attention to more studious observation of the masterpieces. Much to our delight, the wicked sisters prevailed that day.

It was the time that I became aware of my own body. Being the only blond in the family, my mother made it my crowning glory. She loved to brag about her blond daughter and frequently dressed me in red to accentuate the trait. I knew that my parents were sad about my sex, yet they praised me for my feminine attributes creating another insoluble riddle for my child's mind to wrestle with.

I have never been athletic. As I grew into a gangling adolescent, I tried my best to keep up with my older sisters. But, I was never able to master the intricacies of the tire swing, climb a tree or catch a ball like they did, leading to the inevitable conclusion that I was a klutz. That decreased what smidgen of self worth I possessed even more.

Discovering the Monster Within

My father made it a habit of boosting me into the tire swing by grabbing my butt with his hands. Invariably, the action was accompanied by, "Got to give Bustle Butt a hand." He called me Bustle Butt more often than he called me Pat. That was just the kind of encouragement my frail ego needed.

Although photographs of the period contradict my recollection, I perceived my legs as being too stumpy and thick. Perception of one's own body is another thing the anorexic monster distorts. Every mirror I looked into sent back a false impression of my real visage. Anorexics simply cannot see themselves as they really are. This misconception was cruelly reinforced by my parent's second nickname for me, Piano Legs. Even as a young child, I wondered if their cruel nicknames were to embarrass the daughter they didn't want. In the months ahead, I became painfully aware of other parts of my body.

Approaching my seventh birthday, we moved from the Sycamore Street house to Midway. As adults, my sisters and I have discussed the reason for the move. None of us are sure why it transpired. We all believe that it was likely related to Dad's drinking and spending habits. Even with an extra child in the family, we moved from a tidy bungalow into a cracker box cottage with no fresh water in the house.

Moving day remains a vivid memory. The furniture was gone, and Mom was loading us into the car. Our beloved pet, Pumpkin the cat, refused to join us and skillfully stayed just out of reach. We tried coaxing, bribery with her favorite treats and orders in a General Patton command voice. Nothing worked. Disgusted with the cat's behavior, my father ordered us into the car, and we drove away.

Three heartbroken little girls, tears streaming down dusty faces, pressed their noses to the rear window of the car. We watched the image of our beloved Pumpkin grow smaller and smaller as she stood defiantly in the driveway like a lioness guarding her cubs. When she was a tiny speck, I turned away.

I mourned Pumpkin the rest of that summer. Countless times, I was certain that I heard her familiar mew outside or her claws on the back door. Racing to the door, fresh tears flowed each time when Pumpkin wasn't there.

Looking back on it, Pumpkin was trying to tell me something. If I had had any idea of what awaited me at the house on Midway, I would have been better off had I stayed with Pumpkin.

As my father battled his alcoholic addiction to a standstill, a subtle and sinister change occurred in his personality. Admittedly, it was a difficult time for him. After a lifetime of heavy drinking, to stop cold turkey took a monumental effort on his part. But, the sober person he became was in many ways more intolerable for his daughters than the drunk he had been.

For starters, he became even more caustic and critical. My hair was either too long or too short. My dress was always too short. My nails were dirty or needed cut. I talked too much, too loudly, interrupted too often and in general made too much noise. My sisters didn't escape unscathed either. Never a free dispenser of praise or kindness, all traces of either virtue dried up as completely as a desert wash in summer.

During this transformation, I pulled back from him. Accepting his hostility toward me as just punishment for intruding on his idyllic family with my unwanted presence, I felt more isolated, angry and alone than I had before. Turning the emotions inward, I sought refuge in the tire swing my sisters and I had attached to an oak tree in our front yard. There, I tried to make sense of this new man my father had become.

Although it was not overtly manifest, the foundation of my eating disorder was laid at the Sycamore Street table, but it was honed on Midway. Joe Louis was the heavyweight champion of the world then, and the Brown Bomber would have felt right at home at the Archer table during mealtime.

Mealtimes became more contentious as my father crabbed, criticized and berated everyone and everything. Dinner was cold. The meat was either too raw or overdone. All politicians were crooked, and there was no reason to go to church because the only people who did were hypocrites. He was always right, the rest of the world always wrong.

No matter the topic, he reacted the same way. If I didn't eat as much, it served two purposes. Perhaps my bustle butt would go away and my piano legs would melt. Plus, I could escape my father's death-ray mouth more quickly. Food and the table could be used as a weapon. Another tentacle of the multi-armed monster insinuated itself into the fiber of my being and held me close.

In a perfect world, the table should be a calm, happy place where people who love each other sit down to nourish their bodies with food and their spirits with love and comradery. The Archer table was a World War I, Belgian minefield where one false step could spell disaster. The knives at the table were there for cutting the tension as much as for cutting the meat.

The arguments were usually over money, spending habits or children's behavior. Any small incident could trigger a major argument. My sisters and I learned not to say much at mealtime, lest we provide the fuel for another fiery exchange. Although they were violent arguments, no food was ever thrown. It was too expensive to waste, and heaven help a small hand that inadvertently knocked over a glass of milk.

When my father was gone, the tension eased to more tolerable levels, and the table became a happier place where my sisters and I felt more like talking. However, subjects like my father's drinking, could still inadvertently detonate a land mine. We chose peace and avoided those subjects as much as we could.

Mom was sergeant at arms for the family's holy order of thou-shalt-clean-up-thy-plate that was enforced whether my father was home or not. Ungrateful whelps whose eyes were bigger than their bellies were at the mercy of our mother. I cannot begin to guess the number of hours that Linda, sat in front of a plate with peas on it trying to choke them down. Although she hated them, she was forced to take some every time they were cooked, and she was forced to remain at the table until the last one disappeared.

Frequently, a catastrophic event pushes the harried person who is set up for an eating disorder over the edge into the abyss of starvation behavior. As traumatic as mealtimes were, my real catastrophe occurred one night when I was eight. That night, a child's worst nightmare became my way of life. My mother was not at home. Why? I don't remember. My father took me into his bedroom and closed the door. What had I done? What was he going to punish me for? I frantically searched my mind for some offense. I was petrified. I couldn't think of anything.

"It's okay Pat. Just relax. Daddy loves you. Everything will be all right," he cooed with an uncharacteristic huskiness in his voice as he picked me up and laid me gently on the bed.

My heart thudded in my ears like a jackhammer. Slowly, with a peculiar glazed look in his eyes, he pulled my shorts off. Goose bumps of fear and embarrassment dotted my flesh. Next came my panties, and I lay there exposed from the waist down. Shock, revulsion and embarrassment washed over me like a flood tide. I tried to speak, but my throat was so dry only a hoarse croak escaped my lips.

I couldn't comprehend what was happening when I felt his tongue between my legs, over my genitals, up onto my abdomen. What had I done? Oh God, what had I done? This was obviously extreme punishment for some sin I had committed. What was it? Oh God what was it? My stomach churned, and I felt as if I might throw up.

As with most little girls, I had been taught to keep my dress down. I wasn't supposed to let anyone see anything "down there." I wasn't told why, or even where "down there" was for sure. No one ever explained those things to me. I simply knew it was a bad thing to do. Now, I lay naked, defenseless, my father all over me with his tongue and seeming to enjoy my plight as he uttered soft grunts and moans of pleasure. What should I do?

I had no idea how long he continued or exactly what he did. Overwhelmed by the explosion of emotions, sometime during the attack I invoked my talent for disassociation and withdrew into a shell to shut out the horror he was inflicting on me. When I was finally able to focus my thoughts, I was dressed and alone with my guilt and my shame. I didn't understand it. I didn't know what he had done to me or why. I just knew it was something horrible. And, if I didn't know what I had done to cause it, I might accidentally do it again. That night, and on countless others, shaking uncontrollably, I cried myself to sleep.

The brutal attack marked a turning point in my life. My locus of control was disrupted. I was forced to spend the rest of my years at home in fear and terror of being close to or alone with my father. He had stolen my childhood from me. As a result, I never learned to love my father as a daughter should. Neither did I hate him. I simply feared him. Later, when I realized the full scope of what he had done, I became furious with him.

He never was an affectionate man who hugged or kissed us. None of us ever remember sitting on his lap. After the night in his bedroom, I was thankful for that. His usual lack of affection made his actions during the attack even harder for me to understand.

The second attack occurred in the car. My father had an errand to run.

"Pat, why don't you come along with me," he said with a rare warm smile. I immediately agreed. It was a pleasant spring day, and I picked out imagined shapes from the billowing clouds. I enjoyed the ride. I had almost been able to relegate that night in the bedroom to a bad dream.

"Pat, look at me," my father commanded with that unusual huskiness in his voice that propelled me back to the night in his bedroom. My breath stuck in my throat.

With a knot in the pit of my stomach, I turned to look at him, and my eyes widened with shock and surprise. He had his penis out and was fondling it with his free hand. I didn't know that's what you called it, but I knew what it was, thanks to the marble Centurion.

Taking my hand, he placed it on the rigid member and whispered, "Here, honey, feel this. Doesn't that feel nice?"

It *didn't* feel nice! It felt like a hard, revolting worm, and I drew back my hand as if it had been placed on a hot burner. With a cry of revulsion, I scrambled over the seat and into the back. Huddling in the corner tears streamed down my cheeks.

"What the hell's the matter with you?" my father bellowed. "You're gonna break your neck."

This wasn't an isolated incident, and I soon avoided being alone in the car with him. I never again road in the front seat as my fear and embarrassment inched its way closer to anger and hostility.

Lacking running water in our first two houses, our weekly Saturday night baths at Midway were accomplished in a galvanized tub in the middle of the kitchen. After that night in my father's room, each time I climbed naked into the tub, I was in mortal terror that my father would stride into the kitchen and punish me in front of the entire family. I couldn't wait to climb out of the tub and get dressed.

When my father joined A. A., after his Saturday night meetings, we went to family dances. My parents were both excellent dancers, and they taught their girls to dance. Not only our parents but also others who attended taught us too. Since my father was the best dancer, he often assumed the role of instructor.

What should have been a joyous event for a young girl became an approach avoidance conflict for me. My father taught us to love the music and the rhythms. I enjoyed the camaraderie of the loving, giving people who attended those dances. I wanted to be a good daughter who pleased her father by being a great dancer. Maybe if I did, he wouldn't sneak into my room at night to punish me. Instead, I was rigid as a post. I hated it when we danced because he pressed his body so close to mine I could feel his excitement and all the revulsion of those nights roared back to me like a runaway train. Torn by conflicting emotions, I came to dread Saturday nights.

After the abuse began, so did my sleepwalking. The first time, I wandered outside to look for my shoes. Once, when my grandparents were visiting, I went into the living room where they were sitting.

"Pat, honey, what are you doing up?" Grandpa asked me.

"She's asleep, Wally," Grandma said.

"No she isn't. Want some ice cream, Pat?"

"Yes," I answered.

By the time Grandpa Wally came back with the ice cream, I was back in bed, sound asleep, with no recollection of the episode.

My most frightening somnambulating occurred the night I walked out of the front door and around to the back of the house in the middle of the night. My father was at work, and my mother heard the back door rattling as I tried to get back in. Grabbing a baseball bat, she poised at the side of the door ready to bash in the intruder's brain. When I woke up crying, she dropped the bat trembling at the thought of what she might have done to her daughter. I still sleepwalk, but on rare occasion now.

Shortly after my twelfth birthday, my father worked his way up to bookkeeper at Diamond Alkali. Since he no longer drank and gambled, with the raise that accompanied his new job, we could afford a bigger house. As I contemplated our move to Johnny Cake, the conflicts of my childhood escalated. In the new house, we would have indoor plumbing and running water for the first time in my life. But, with the extra rooms, there would be more places I could be trapped by my father. Maybe if I was thinner, I would be harder for him to find.

As I reflect on it, my father was sly. Although I had no way of knowing it, he was abusing all three of us at the same time. I never found out about my sisters until I was an adult. None of us knew about the others. How he was able to do that without the others of us knowing, in houses that were so small, was diabolically clever. Another obvious question, did my mother know about it?

My sisters and I have discussed it, and we agree. If she knew, she never gave a hint of it to any of us. Retrospectively, I wonder if she at least suspected something. She developed a sudden, unusual interest in church. It was almost as if she was trying to separate us from him in some ways. Did she think our involvement in religion might give us the courage we needed to resist? Was that the reason she frequently leaped to our defense when he attacked us verbally? Was it part of the reason their relationship was filled with rancor? I will never be able to answer those questions, since I didn't ask them of my mother before she died. That will forever haunt me.

I know that my mother loved me, and would have given her life to protect me. A child looks to its mother for nurture, for guidance and for protection. My child's heart of hearts cries out, "Why didn't you know? Where were you? Why didn't you protect me?" For her sake, I hope that she never knew, but if she did, God has given me the compassion to forgive her.

My father, my sisters and I, and probably our mother, each had a secret, and secrets can sometimes be painful. We hid, ignored, buried and kept secret the most dreadful things. It made it easier for me to hide the monster when it engulfed me later in life. It's the way my family dealt with things. It's how I learned to handle adversity. We never talked out a problem. We yelled, argued, fought, berated, got sarcastic, or more often buried the unresolved discord where it smoldered like compost in a heap turning everything to decay. That training made it easy for me to hide the monster in later years.

How did I, or does any child for that matter, survive such a horror? My situation is not unique. Since I have found the courage to speak of my abuse, a surprising number of women have shared similar stories with me. Each of us had our own defense mechanisms. They were similar in kind but unique to the survivor. If the defenses are flawed, the victim is consumed by guilt, shame and grief. If they are strong, the child survives, but not without scars that no one can see.

The victim in the box I had become accepted the attacks as punishment for some unknown atrocity that I must have committed. I wasn't worthy to be part of the family. Was this the cost of staying a part of it? This was exactly what I deserved, and I should accept it and be quiet about it.

I survived by detaching myself from the act itself, blotting most of it from my conscious memory. I was a bystander, too frightened and ashamed to be an unwilling participant. That's why the details of my assaults are a blur. I simply don't remember exactly what happened.

Discovering the Monster Within

As I examine it rationally, could things have happened that I would swear never did? Of course they could have. To think that he repeatedly assaulted me over seven years without deriving any pleasure for himself defies logic. Would remembering the exact details of the events be of value to my healing? I don't know, but I doubt it. To learn more sordid details wouldn't change how I feel about what happened, and the defenses allowed me to survive and form a healthy attitude toward sex as an adult. Though some therapists might disagree, I think I should leave well enough alone. I don't need all the gory details.

The assaults continued into my early teens. Why did they go on so long? First, I felt totally worthless, so anything that he did to me couldn't make me feel any worse about myself.

Besides, I knew that somehow I was responsible for what he did to me. I was responsible for his behavior, not him. And, if I made too much trouble, they might expel me from the family. Then what would I do?

A combination of events ended the abuse, and it started with the church. Aside from the reasons mentioned earlier, church gave my mother a way to escape the miseries of her daily life as well. That was the thing that motivated our new involvement in religion. It became a hideout for the Archer women.

Mom was in charge of the church kitchen and my sisters and I pulled K.P. duty for most of the church dinners and social functions. And, we had a ball. In that place, filled with love and kindness, we forgot our petty squabbles and surrendered to the joy of it all. I recall how sad I felt when the last pot was scrubbed, the last dish dried, and we had to go home.

When I was thirteen, I went to the Methodist Youth Fellowship Camp at Lakeside, Ohio. It is a wonderful place on the shores of Lake Erie, but it was my first trip away from home by myself. Despite my hectic home life, I felt homesick. But, I soon got over it.

During that week, I made my first real acquaintance with God, and found a more important reason to go to church. It was connected to Psalm 22:1. I memorized the verse because it so fit my life.

Pull the Trigger

"My God, my God, why hast thou forsaken me?"

Jesus cried those words from the cross. If the Son of God could feel that way, it gave me hope that I could somehow find salvation from a life that seemed so futile. That week cemented my foundation in a life-long walk with God. When he learned of it, my father found the whole thing perverse.

At the same time, an important person entered my life in the form of Reverend Leonard Budd, who was our youth pastor. Pastor Len was the first adult in my life who ever accepted me as a person of worth with a head on my shoulders. He was also the first man in my life who didn't view me as a scatter-brained reproduction machine. I could talk to him, and he listened to me.

I felt comfortable and at peace when I was at the church. I saw more kindness from the people who worshiped there than I ever believed could exist. I know I was grasping at anything to get out of the house. I had few other friends, and the church became the focus of my social life.

One thing anorexics do is to put down or minimize praise or personal accomplishment. A compliment denies our worthless perception of ourselves. I showed that trait long before the monster completely took hold of me. I was elected president of our youth fellowship group, and even now have difficulty writing about it. The victim in me still tells me I didn't deserve the honor. Fortunately, I don't listen to the victim any more.

In my capacity as president, I had a lot of contact with Pastor Len, and we became friends. If any of us needed a ride home after our meetings, he obliged. Since I *always* needed one, we had a lot of time to talk as he drove me home. He was a great listener and never tired of my complaints about home, school or family. Although I probably had a teenaged crush on the gentle man, he never knew it, and I remember our relationship as my first, true, adult friendship.

Since he was so important to me at the time, I talked about him a lot at home. Occasionally, he called me or I called him about MYF business. It raised my father's ire. Although he didn't attack Pastor Len personally, the general attacks against the church and those who served as its leaders became more vitriolic. Mom invited Pastor Len to dinner on occasion, and I loved to watch my father squirm. Was he afraid I might expose our dirty little secret to my new friend? He needn't have worried. I never did. Guilt, shame and fear froze me. I could never talk about it with anyone until the last few years.

Another important cog in the machine that allowed me to end the assaults surrounded my 4H project that summer. The club was a wonderful experience and Mrs. Eisenburg, our leader, taught me many things. I entered a red jumper that I had made in the fashion contest and won! As a reward, I was invited to model my creation in the big show. I still remember how my knees knocked as I shyly walked among the crowd. It was the first time I had ever been the center of attention like that. I find it difficult to recount how it made me feel. For the first time, I realized that I was somebody, who could do something on my own and be successful. Unfortunately, the lesson didn't stick.

Work also added to the courage I needed to find to end things. I started baby sitting at age nine and was never without some sort of job. When I was older, along with my sisters, I boarded the trucks that took us to the nearby farmer's orchards and fields to pick peaches, apples, cherries or strawberries. The work was hard and the pay small, but I loved it. Later on, I worked for a dry-cleaning establishment and in a soda fountain as a soda jerk. The jerk part gave my few friends material for a plethora of playful jabs.

It was also at the time that I realized that I wanted to be a nurse. It is not unusual to find an anorexic in a helping profession. Since the major issue in the anorexic's life is control, what better job than to be a nurse. I might not be able to control my own life, but on the nursing unit, my word would be law, my orders would be obeyed, and I would be in complete charge. I told my father about it.

"I want to go to college and be a nurse," I began hesitantly.

Looking down his narrow nose at me, disgust contorted his features and he said, "What the hell for? If you think I'm gonna waste a cent of my money sending you to college, you're nuts! Even if you go, you'll just get married, have a house full of kids and not work anyhow. Forget that nonsense!"

Turning away, he walked out of the room, and I fled to the sanctity of my bedroom where I made a vow that I would go to school no matter what. I was earning money of my own. I pledged to immediately open my own savings account and to save half of all the money I earned for school. His denial helped me realize that if I really wanted to go to school, I couldn't depend on him. I would have to do it on my own.

During this time, I developed such negativity about life and myself that I began to think, dream and fanaticize about death. What would it be like to be dead? Would it be quiet and peaceful or would I still hear my father's strident criticism? Would it be nothingness? Would the pain and humiliation go away?

Sinking deeper into my self-constructed well of depression, I had a great deal of difficulty falling asleep and then slept fitfully. Although I occasionally walked in my sleep, it was infrequent. On those nights when sleep wouldn't come, as I lay there in the darkness terrified that my father would open the bedroom door, I began to fantasize disasters.

What if my legs were gone? What if I were paralyzed, or blind? What if I were critically ill? Would he leave me alone then? Only when I could visualize that some catastrophe had befallen me, and that I had gotten what I deserved, could I fall into a troubled sleep. My favorite was blindness. In the total darkness, I felt I might find peace. If not, at least I wouldn't be able to see him coming.

I realize now, that I was trying to regain control of my life. If I were the blighted one, the object of attention, I could bring him to me on my terms, and I'd be in control again. It was all about control, and I didn't have any.

By now, my father was coming into my room once or twice a month. Each time I felt a deepening sense of guilt and shame and compensated by dwelling on the dark side and disassociating myself from him. Running away became a daily fantasy. I firmly believe that these late adolescent early teen years of negativity and self-loathing affected my entire life. It plowed the field so the monster could sew its seed in fertile ground.

Then, if it was possible, a worse thing happened that filled me with terror and convinced me that these episodes were unholy. As I entered my teenage years, gradually, I began to feel excitement and even pleasure from his assaults. Before, I had been able to escape completely from the physical sensations. Now, God help me, I was almost looking forward to his predatory visitations.

The intricate pieces aligned on my fourteenth birthday when my father presented me with a beautiful colored glass bracelet. I remember the way the light made the tiny glass beads flash as if they possessed their own internal fire.

More remarkable was the gift itself. It was not the sort of thing any of us ever got.

I can still hear the "Wow, look at that!" from Beverly. "Oooh, how lucky you are," from Linda. And, our father had given it to me. He never gave gifts so personal or frivolous. Why this never raised red flags with my sisters or my mother, I have no idea. I believe it should have with my mother. If it did, she gave no indication.

Looking across the table at him, I could see the subtle signs on his face, and I knew at once the reason for the bauble. It was a bribe! I truly believe he could sense my conflict between guilt and pleasure, and he was bribing me to choose pleasure. Shame overwhelmed me, and I could almost hear Pastor Len's voice condemning me for the sinner I was. If I took that bracelet, and allowed the attacks to continue, I was nothing but a harlot!

Fixing on the rainbow of hues from the sparkling bracelet, I said to myself, "You will never touch me again!"

Out loud, I said, "Thank you. It's lovely."

My sisters never understood why I wasn't overjoyed with the gift and didn't dance around the table with joy.

Pull the Trigger

Two nights later, the door to my room opened softly, and he came up to the edge of my bed. For the very first time, I wasn't terrified. I was mad as hell.

Crabbing back to the far corner of the mattress, I found my voice and hissed like a viper, "No more! Don't touch me! Don't you ever dare touch me again! Don't you ever come near me again! *Ever!*"

He hesitated. Then coming closer, he reached for me, and I batted at his hand saying, "If you touch me, I'll scream! I'll scream my lungs out, and you'll have to explain to all of them why you're here."

His instant temper flared, and even in the dark I could feel his eyes boring into me with a fierceness that I knew was hatred. Gaining a modicum of control, he managed to turn and leave the room without one of his characteristic outbursts.

After the first time, my father never spoke to me during an assault. I thought then, and believe in my heart now, that he never recognized me as a person. I was just a thing, an outlet for his ravenous sexual appetite that he was impotent to satisfy in an acceptable adult fashion. Realizing that did nothing for my self esteem. Even in the face of my defiance, he couldn't bring himself to speak to me.

He came back one more time with the same result. Convinced I would raise the entire house if he came anywhere near me again, he never came back to my room. Unfortunately, the hatred and animosity it engendered stressed the tortured dynamics of the Archer house nearly to the breaking point.

From that day on, the public relationship between my father and me rivaled the current relationship between North and South Korea. Every conversation was filled with tension between two people with different ideologies. I didn't dream it possible, but his criticism of me turned more vicious. After that, I don't think I ever did anything that ever pleased him. He challenged everything I said and everything I did. The most innocent comment on my part was reason for him to launch a scathing tirade.

Discovering the Monster Within

Sensing the level of tension, my mother felt it her mission to defend me against him with even more vigor than she had pursued in the past. It makes me wonder if she knew what was going on, and it gave her more courage to oppose him. I can't be sure. Regardless, the combination of circumstances made the rest of my days at home nearly unbearable.

CHAPTER 4

Siblings, Pets, and Other Disasters

hildren develop rolls within the family unit. Traditionally, the firstborn is the hero. This child gets the good grades; succeeds most of the time regardless of the endeavor; seems to handle most everything and bends over backward to please their parents.

My oldest sister, Beverly, had a large frame like my grandfather. At five feet eight, she weighed more than me most of the time. Although she was an average student, she was aggressive, good in sports and a real tomboy. Unfortunately, girls were not encouraged to do such things in the late nineteen forties. Sharing that interest with my father, she was closer to him than the rest of us. With that closeness came a terrible price that she eventually paid. This unfortunate relationship blunted her emotional growth and voided her opportunity to become a typical first child. It also left her with her own eating disorder that was the opposite of mine. Beverly was a chronic overeater her entire life.

In a normal family, since the first child gets the lion's share of the attention and praise, a second child typically settles for negative attention and becomes the rebel. Again, the Archer girls refused to fit the mold. Linda was the peacemaker; the arbitrator; the compliant one who would do anything to keep the peace. Unfortunately for her, that was an impossible task in our family.

Linda was the tiny sister at five feet three, with a small frame. She only weighed ninety-nine pounds when she got married. And, that was without the help of any eating disorder. Always the compliant one, she tried her best to please both of my parents, no matter how unreasonable they were. Life, and my father, battered her down to the point that she has a difficult time asserting herself. She'd rather suffer quietly than stick up for what she wants. She is the only one of us without an eating disorder.

In the early years, we did the usual things girls do. Paper dolls, jump rope and jacks were among the favorite games we played. I wasn't very good at the physical games, but I loved them just the same. As we got older, our divergent personalities became a source of friction.

We fought over the temperature; who was supposed to do dishes; whose clothes were junking the room; you name it, we fought over it. As is common when there are three in a dispute, it was always two against one. When two of us disagreed, the third sister leaped into the fray on one side or the other. Fortunately, it was not always the same sister and not always the same side. Thank goodness for that.

Rarely did our disagreements turn physical, but one episode stands out for me. My sisters and I were peeling potatoes, and one of our customary squabbles erupted. I don't remember what it was about, but I was really getting under Linda's skin. The angrier she became, the more I turned the screw. Finally, I pushed her over the edge, and she abandoned her role of peacemaker. Grabbing a larger spud, Linda launched a fastball at my head. She didn't have good aim, and Pat the klutz didn't react quickly enough, and I caught the tuberous missile with my gut. Ouch! It knocked the wind right out of me. When I recovered, I felt bad about the incident. Since I was the instigator, the victim inside assured me that I got exactly what I deserved.

On Sycamore, my sisters and I shared one bedroom, and I slept in the same bed as my sister, Linda. The first bed I remember was a four-poster and still holds a fond spot in my heart. My worldly elder sisters taught me that if I carefully placed today's chewing gum strategically on one of the bedposts, it would retain enough flavor and elasticity for another days chewing. Such tips were practical in a family where such frivolities as gum were a rarity.

On Midway, which was a smaller house, the three of us continued to share a bedroom. Bev had a twin bed while Linda and I shared bunk beds. Being the smallest, she got the top bunk. What few clothes we owned were stored in two boxes beneath the bed. Two hooks on the wall allowed us to hang longer items, like winter coats.

By the time we moved to Johnny Cake, my father had stopped drinking so we were able to afford a slightly larger house. Extra room meant new sleeping arrangements. Beverly, who was twelve years older than Dave, shared a bedroom with him. Linda and I shared a double bed in the second while our parents had their own bedroom again.

The reason I mention the sleeping arrangements is to underscore how really cleaver my father was with his abuse. He was abusing all three of us, and none of us knew the other was being assaulted. How could he have done that? I have spent hours trying to make sense of it, and I can't. I don't think we were particularly dense. Perhaps we were all in denial, or was it that he was so diabolic about the whole thing?

Our first two houses lacked indoor plumbing, and we had the traditional four rooms and path. Indoor plumbing wasn't part of my life until my teenage years. At night, and in defense against the frigid winter winds that scream mercilessly across Lake Erie to batter this northeast corner of Ohio, we had a chamber pot. The cold rim of that pot on my bare bottom is another souvenir of my childhood.

Cold has always been anathema to me. But, I will never forget the paralyzing snow storm of November, nineteen fifty that dropped several feet of snow on the Eastern United States. It was one of the more frightening experiences of my childhood.

Discovering the Monster Within

My father was trapped at work and couldn't get home. There was not enough food in the house to last till he got home. So, when the larders were depleted, mom bundled us up, and we set off for the store.

The storm had cleared the sky to that cobalt blue that is so cherished during long Lake Erie winters. With it came the plunging temperatures and the cold that ate through my clothes and mittens boring into the core of me like a knife made of ice. Despite my resemblance to an Eskimo on the tundra, I shivered from the cold.

Snowdrifts seemed like mountains as mom broke through the waist high drifts that the wind had formed since the plow had been down the street. Thinking of anything that would take my mind off the snow, I was jolted back to reality when my mother screamed.

Mom had tangled in her long coat and fallen awkwardly into the deep snow. It cascaded over her prostrate form, and she disappeared from sight. The three of us were frantic, while Dave, who was too little to understand, simply cried.

Shrieking and wailing, we called to her and dug frantically with our hands while she tried to right herself. It seemed like forever until we cleared some snow away, and she was able to get back onto her feet. Tears of relief froze on our cheeks as we hugged her fiercely.

Standing on that frozen street, I felt the guilt creep into the victim's box where I lived. If I hadn't been an extra mouth to feed there would have been enough supplies to outlast the storm. Mom would never have gone out in the freezing cold, and none of this would have happened. How much longer would they let me stay in this family? Turning the emotions in as I always did, they rooted, festered and haunted me.

When we finally got indoor plumbing, we had a septic system that presented its share of problems. But, we were so overjoyed to at last have indoor plumbing, that even my father was able to forgive the occasional backup, after his usual string of expletives and fit of temper of course. It also gave our father another reason to berate us as the cause for any malodorous malfunctions.

Siblings, Pets, and Other Disasters

One might imagine, with three teenaged daughters, a single bathroom could be a potential source of conflict. It wasn't. We were so thrilled with the convenience it represented, that we willingly shared it. It wasn't unusual to find one of us on the commode, another in the tub and the third curling her hair at the sink. Regardless of the other battles we fought, a truce was always in effect when we needed to share the bath.

The foundation in the weed-choked lot next to us on Sycamore Street is another source of fond memories. Since we lacked the tangible things of childhood, my sisters and I were forced to exercise our imaginations for entertainment. As a result, we gave those imaginations permission to run rampant. The innocent collection of bricks, that was a neighborhood eyesore, became Cinderella's Castle, Black Beard's pirate ship, and any other place the three of us could imagine.

In the summer, wild flowers grew in abundance among the dandelions and broom sage.

The colors never failed to bring a smile to my lips, and I can still smell the fragrance that emanated from that field. It provided the perfume for my regal apparel when Prince Charming invited me to dinner. It was a place of wonder. A place to flee the realities of life and immerse myself into a make believe world where I could feel loved and accepted. Feeling unloved and unaccepted at home, those fantasies helped me to escape reality for a little while.

At the Midway house, a plethora of ancient hardwood trees populated the spacious grounds. One of them perpetually contained a rope and tire swing, that replaced our vacant lot as the fuel for my fantasies. Swinging high into the sky, I allowed my imagination to soar and left my fears, pain and loneliness on the earth below.

The back of that house contained an external entrance to the basement. Slanted doors that opened like a book fascinated me. At one time, it may have been a coal chute. I was never sure about that. Despite my curiosity with the doors, I cannot remember ever being in that basement. The memory is so vivid; I can't imagine that I never went in there. I wonder if I did but for some reason have blocked out the memories. I never had the courage to pose the question to my father. Now, I'm not sure I want to know.

There was never enough money to go round, so my mother went to work in a doll factory. Once a year, my sisters and I were allowed to go to the factory with her and choose a doll each from the rejects that failed quality control inspection. Though they were considered flawed by the experts, to us they were treasures.

Our poverty level income affected us in other ways. Two episodes remain clear in my memory. One involved mom's mangle iron. While playing with my sisters while mom ironed, I inadvertently put my hand on the board as mom brought the hot metal iron down. The pain caused me to scream in agony as my hand burned.

She couldn't afford to take me to the doctor so Mom came to the rescue again. She treated it with tender loving care and a poultice of tea leaves. Fortunately, it healed without scars. I clearly remember the dichotomy of the excruciating pain in my hand and the tenderness and loving care of my mother as she soothed me and changed the bandages.

Since I was not blessed with strong teeth, dental hygiene has always been crucial to me. A tooth rotted when I was eight, and mom took me to the dentist. He pulled the tooth without numbing it. Tears streamed down my face when I came out of his office. When my mother found out what had happened, she stormed past the receptionist and into the doctor's office where she read him the riot act.

Standing in the office, the pattern that was even then already a way of life, was reinforced. The entire situation was my fault. If I had been tougher, stronger, I wouldn't have cried and Mom wouldn't have gotten upset with the dentist. Why was I always so much trouble for her?

Although things were difficult, I have some pleasant memories of my childhood. Despite working, taking care of the house and raising four children, Mom still tried to make things fun for us. There was a park near the Midway house, and when she could find time, she packed a picnic lunch for us, and we had a feast in the park. It quickly became our new magic kingdom to replace the foundation we left on Sycamore Street.

Since there was no drinking water, we hauled it in once a week from a source about a mile away. Mom even tried to make the drudgery fun. Most of the time, she succeeded, except in the fierce heat of summer or the biting cold of winter.

She did the same with holidays. On my seventh birthday, she made me a Maypole using long strips of cloth. She explained the tradition of the spring festival, and my sisters and I danced around the festive standard like shameless Druids.

One Christmas tradition I remember with particular fondness. On December seventh, my sisters and I would write a letter to Santa. I was not a precocious child, preferring to remain out of the limelight lest I become more of a problem. Mom helped me write when I was too young. On a cold night soon after, Mom would build a roaring fire in the great room, and we burned the letters, sending the smoke up our great brick chimney with our wishes to Santa Heaven.

There was always a Christmas tree, with pretty lights, garlands and shinny ornaments of the variety that made little hearts beat with excitement and anticipation. Mom decorated the fireplace and the windowsills, turning our day-to-day great room into a magical place where elves might be real.

We were taught early the joys of practicality. Christmas was a time when the Archer sisters stocked up on much needed items. New winter coats, hats, boots, mittens, underwear and pajamas were the order of the day. To some children, used to a cornucopia of toys, this would have resulted in upturned noses. To us, they were each special treasures.

Despite the physical limitations of the house, I have many wonderful memories of my time at Midway. I remember helping my mother mix the yellow block of food coloring into the amorphous lump of white goo that became margarine. To my child's imagination, that was magic.

Another culinary treat was rendering bits of pork rind into crisp, tasty, grease-laden yummies that we coated with salt and ate instead of the potato chips we couldn't afford. Later, when my monster held complete sway, I physically gagged when I remembered those artery-hardening treats I had coveted as a child. Even though I am well on my way to recovery, I have no plans to fry up a batch for friends and family any time soon.

Excluding the foods just mentioned, I have noticed that those foods my mind remembers fondly from my childhood are the one ones I have the hardest time reintroducing to my diet. Things like mashed potatoes carry a double whammy since that was one of the foods I used in my binge-purge cycles.

Both my parents smoked, and with the cost of ready-made cigarettes, they rolled their own. With today's spiraling cost of cigarettes, we are nearly back to those times. They used an old-fashioned drum roller, and even the family klutz, became a competent cigarette maker. I loved these weekly sessions because they were happy, harmonious times when animosity, anger, bickering and sarcasm were suspended. My father stayed relatively sober, and we behaved like a normal family for a few hours.

Whenever we were able to get a few extra pennies, we used the money to buy yarn to make dolls that in turn we sold to earn spending money. The extra funds allowed us to buy a few things that would otherwise have been beyond our reach.

Shortly after moving to Midway, our annual trips to the enchanted island began. Grandpa Schilpp owned an island with a cabin in Canada. Once a year my sisters and I squirmed with anticipation as we watched the hands of the clock snail around its face until it was time for my father to come home from work. While he cleaned up and changed, we packed the car and were off to Canada. It didn't take long for the adrenalin rush to be overwhelmed by the late hour and the hum of the tires on the pavement. When we awoke, we were there!

Perched on a rise, the T-shaped shingled bungalow with large, awning shaded windows, surrounded by a lake, was the scene of some of my happiest childhood moments. A curved path, lined with stones, wound its way between tall thin pines to the dock. Wooden folding chairs for sitting and sunning rested near the end of the twelve foot long wooden platform.

Grandpa's boat was moored at the end of the dock in shallow enough water for little girls to wade and play. When we learned to swim, deeper water was near by. The diminutive row boat was a grand yacht where we entertained royalty, a pirate ship where we were held prisoner by Captain Kid, a Mississippi river boat where we sang and danced to adoring fans or a fishing platform where Grandpa taught us the rudiments of the sport.

The cool shade of the island provided ample room for us to run and play and dream. It was an oasis from poverty, overcrowding, tension, assaults by my father and the strife of daily life. Unfortunately, the time flew by when we were there, and all too soon, it was back to reality. The vacations ended forever when he sold the island in the mid-fifties.

We had few contacts with other relatives. My father had no living kin so all my memories are of Mom's folks. Grandpa Walter (Wally) Schilpp taught at West Technical High in Cleveland. His hobby was building houses. Once he had completed my Grandma's dream house, she would find something wrong with it. With a shrug of his broad shoulders, he'd begin planning a new house. When it was done, they'd sell the one they lived in and moved to the new one where the cycle would begin again.

Since grandpa nearly always had a current construction site, they made great places to play. We liked to wind the curled wood shavings into our hair to make Scarlet O'Hara curls. Grandpa's patience with our squealing, giggling interference stood in stark contrast to our father's impatience.

The only other relatives who ever visited were my mom's sister, Aunt Ellie, and her second husband Uncle John. Her first husband had been killed in the Battle of the Bulge. They had a son, Johnnie, who was a two-year-old terrorist. My major memory of that encounter was a painful one. The little brat bit my big toe, leaving me in pain for days.

Discovering the Monster Within

My relationship with my brother, Dave, was tainted by a number of things over the years. First, he was the boy they wanted, and for the first five years after Dave was born, I expected any day to find my bags packed and sitting on the front porch with a note instructing me to leave the family. When I was finally able to get over that, I tried to treat him as any big sister treats her little brother, but we never were particularly close.

Part of the reason was the way my father treated him. Dave was a boy, thus exempt from non-manly chores. He was placed on his own little pedestal and was subject to an entirely different set of rules. I'm glad for that. Maybe he has less unpleasant memories of childhood than my sisters and I do.

For example, the only social events we attended regularly were Dave's baseball games. As many fathers do, my father tried to recapture his own missed opportunities through his child. Tragically, the scene is repeated every day at little league fields or arenas in every sport. A parent, never good enough to make a team themselves, or with dreams of pro sports mega- contracts dancing in their heads, mercilessly push a ten year old far beyond his or her own abilities. That's what my father did to Dave

Dave, by his own admission not a good athlete, tried his best, but it was never good enough. Even when they practiced, my father was constantly shouting, criticizing, berating. Fortunately, he didn't carry that attitude over to the rest of Dave's life.

Since Dave's athletic prowess was so important to my father, it became a family priority, and we were all compelled to go not only to his games but even his practice sessions. Despite the negative aura surrounding the situation, there were positive things about it, too.

It was a time when my father wasn't focused on my sisters and me, providing us with a respite from his criticisms. Mom always baked cookies or brought sugared doughnut holes for us to enjoy. It was no surprise that she was a favorite of the other players and coaches.

These visits to the ballpark remained a focus long after I left home. I remember returning from nursing school for a visit and being ordered to grab a bite so we could get to Dave's game. According to my sister, Dave hates baseball as a result, and I can certainly understand why. But, my sisters and I enjoyed those times of freedom and the opportunity to be out of the house.

I think another reason Dave and I never were able to be close was a fallout from my father's abuse of me. From the day I put a stop to the abuse, the relationship between my father and me was extremely strained as I mentioned earlier.

Since I only publicly acknowledged the abuse as an adult, and subsequently discovered the abuse of my sisters, Dave was oblivious to it. As a result, the only thing he saw was the conflict between our father and me, and he blamed me for it.

"Why did you always have to antagonize, Dad?" he has asked me as an adult. "You were always causing trouble, playing the holier than thou role. Everything he said, you took exception to. You were the cause of all the trouble at home."

At the time he said it, I was still too much of a victim to disagree. I still feel bad about the situation. Despite how he feels about me, I love my brother. The victim in me still wants to take the blame. If I had told the rest of the family what was happening, Dave might have understood. If I had just kept quiet and not allowed my anger with my father to turn to hate, it might have been better.

But, the victim is no longer in the box. I know that nothing I could have done would have tempered the hostility in my father's tortured brain. Nothing I could have done, then, would have made Dave understand. He was too young. As an adult, I pray he would be Christian enough to understand what I went through and realize that I was not the shrew he pictured me to be. Only after I had been to Remuda, did I find the courage to be more aggressive in resolving this issue with him. Until then, I just couldn't fight for myself because of my rotten self-esteem. I didn't think I was worth fighting for. Mustering my courage, I emailed Dave and bared my soul to him. Fortunately, he answered me, and we have opened a dialogue to settle our differences.

Discovering the Monster Within

My sisters and I didn't have a lot of friends. On Johnny Cake, our next-door neighbors, the Mahoney's, raised horses. Although we were never close enough friends to be invited over for a ride, I still loved to watch the stately animals prance around the field, their heads held high, and manes flowing in the wind. They supplied the fuel for a thousand daydreams, and I made good use of them.

Since my parents weren't particularly friendly people, we barely knew the people on the other side of us either. But, behind us lived the Eisenburgs, and their daughters Doris and Gayle became life long friends for Linda and me.

They were only slightly better off financially than we were, and were the kindest people I can remember from my childhood. They never made an issue of financial things. Both girls had bicycles, something we could never hope for. But, they always shared them with us. Sometimes, we would simply take turns riding up and down a quiet street. Other times, Linda and Doris might use them while Gayle and I did other things, or vice versa.

The four of us frittered away happy hours playing ball, swinging on vines in a nearby ravine, or laying on our backs daydreaming in the sunshine. On Halloween, trick or treat was a shared event, as was window soaping and eating candy, something I enjoyed then.

Over the years, Gayle became one of my best friends and remained so until her untimely death. She always accepted me for the way I was, fat, acne scarred and clumsy, as I saw myself, never holding any of it against me. She only saw *me*, and liked me for that alone. I'll always be grateful to her for that.

Despite our financial circumstances, there was a never-ending series of pets around the house. Dogs, cats, rabbits and gerbils, you name it. A veritable menagerie of animals spiced up my childhood. Pumpkin, the stray calico, with a mind of her own who refused to move, was my constant companion while we lived on Sycamore Street.

Our dog, Topper, was our favorite pet on Midway. We got him during the snowstorm of nineteen fifty. The lady, who sold him to us as at a bargain basement price, assured us that he was pure cocker spaniel. As he grew older, and the wirehair, chin whiskers and black and brown spots appeared, we realized she had been less than truthful. It didn't matter. We loved him anyway. Besides, mom said all the dogs we owned were Heinz dogs, fifty-seven varieties.

That dog was involved in two traumatic events at the Archer house. One day, my sister Linda was wrestling on the bed with the dog when he was a puppy, and Topper bit her lip resulting in a laceration. I distinctly remember the dread I felt about what my father might do when he came home. If only I had taken the dog outside to play, I could have prevented my sister's pain and saved Topper from my father's wrath.

Topper survived the ordeal, but my father cursed and screamed and beat the poor animal until I was sure he wouldn't live through it. During my father's tirade, I cowered in the corner trying to be as small as possible lest I be the next victim of his wrath. Every time something happened in my universe, it revolved around me. It was my, fault somehow. I could have prevented the disaster. It took me most of my life to realize that wasn't true.

Although I was already good at accepting the victim's role, I was truly culpable in the second episode involving Topper. When he came to live with us, we already had a cat named, Dolly. The enmity between the two of them was classic for their species.

Each morning, when we left for school, it was our job to put the cat outside and to tie Topper, who was still a pup, so he wouldn't soil the house or chew up the furniture. Mom and Dad were at work, and Dave was with the babysitter. Up late, we dashed around the house fighting over the washbasin, throwing together breakfast and in general creating chaos. With time running out, we dashed out the door and down the path to the road.

"Pat, did you tie Topper?" Linda asked me.

"I thought you did," I said defensively.

"Well, I didn't," Linda answered in a tone I interpreted as accusatory. The victim had screwed up again.

Discovering the Monster Within

Turning with tears of embarrassment in my eyes, I tore back to the house, dragged Topper to the kitchen and lashed him to the bottom drawer of the stove where mom kept her skillets. It was his usual tether. Hurrying out the door, I ran to catch my sisters.

When we came home after an uneventful day at school, we walked up to the door. It banged open and the cat and the dog flew from the house spitting and yelping. We cowered at the edge of the yard afraid to go inside. Finally, we worked up enough courage to go inside.

The house looked as if a cyclone had slipped in through the keyhole and decimated the interior. Tables were overturned, skillets littered the floor, and a lamp lay in shards. Every cushion was off every piece of furniture and scattered on the floor. Not a single room was spared. The three of us began to wail in unison as our father screamed obscenities.

I forgot to put out the cat! The hound from hell had dragged the drawer from the stove around the house ricocheting off doorframes and furniture like a ping-pong ball. Our father ranted on for what seemed like an eternity while we quaked in terror. And, all of it was my fault!

Fighting the urge to hide under the bed, we waited for our sentence to be passed like prisoners before the bar. Our father, resembling a red-faced ogre, meted out the punishment. Even though we were certain that this would be the exception to the rule, it wasn't. By the time he was finished using words like, stupid, ungrateful, irresponsible and careless, he may as well have removed the outer layers of our skin. We were sentenced to clean up the house, a chore that took the remainder of the day and well into the evening.

The whole episode was my fault. I didn't let the cat out. Why was he punishing my sisters too?

One of the more traumatic events of my childhood involved another dog. On the street in front of our house, a car hit another of our dogs, but the impact didn't kill it. The poor creature writhed and whined pitifully in mortal agony on the pavement, its back broken.

"Go to the house and bring me a pan of water from the pump," my father commanded.

"What for?" I asked through my tears.

"Just shut up and do it!" he screamed at me.

Racing to the house, I complied with the order, and while my sisters and I watched in horror, our father added to the poor creature's misery by trying to drown it with the water. Still, the valiant creature refused to die.

In desperation, my father called the police who ended the dog's misery with a bullet. Fortunately, the police spared us the final act of cruelty and sent us to the house. We heard the gunshot from there. That was the first time I wondered what it might be like to be dead. I wouldn't be a problem to anyone, if I were dead.

Animals were abundant at Johnny Cake also. Besides the usual dogs, we had a three-legged cat mom named Sammy as well as gerbils and hamsters. Since my father loved birds, an assortment of parakeets, lovebirds and other small, feathered things swooped constantly about the house.

Sammy deserves special note. After the first litter of kittens, we changed *her* name to Samantha. Mom joked that having three legs didn't interfere with her social life. I identified with that cat. I was damaged goods, just like Samantha. If she could make a normal life for herself, maybe I could, too.

Because of my father's volatile temper, one event from our childhood stands out. Once, when my sister, Linda, ran away, Beverly and I ran around the house hiding everything we could think of that might be used to whip her. We needn't have bothered. She was never spanked. Despite the physical violence with my mother, and nearly everyone else in his world, he rarely physically punished any of us. He knew why Linda ran away, and if he was too harsh with her, she might have revealed her secret. He couldn't afford that.

A rare case of corporal punishment involved a broken window. There was disagreement between the three of us as to who the actual culprit was. As a result, none of us would confess or point out the guilty party.

Our recalcitrance drove our father into a frenzy. The three of us were laid across the bed and summarily spanked.

The broken window allowed another opportunity for me to play the victim. Even though I wasn't sure who broke the window, if I hadn't done it, it at least was my fault that it got broken. I wanted to confess, but was too scared to do it. Would my sisters ever forgive me?

Not long after we moved to Johnny Cake, we got a small television. Since all things in the house resolved around our father, the television set was no different. He told us when the set could be on and what we could watch. Nothing was allowed to interfere with baseball or football or whatever else struck his fancy.

One of the programs that we were required to watch each Saturday evening was The Lawrence Welk Show. I realize that Mr. Welk is a show business legend, but, my father's attitude turned the program into an ordeal, and I was never able to appreciate Mr. Welk's genius.

Occasionally, he would fall asleep during a program, and we would sneak to the television and try to quietly change the channel. Most of the time, he woke up. When he did, we quickly flipped the channel back to the original program and scampered from the room like mine rats before a cave in.

Mom changed a lot too. Entering a premature change of life, she was perpetually tired. There was ample reason for her fatigue. Besides trying to be a good mother to us, she taught sewing, worked at the doll factory, and sold Avon.

I remember an occasion when she cut herself in the kitchen while cooking dinner. It was the kind of small laceration every cook has experienced, but she was so exhausted that she uncharacteristically started to cry and fainted. Of course, my father interpreted it as a classic example of the weakness of the female of the species.

Mom was a good teacher, but as she aged her patience wore thin. Besides sewing, cooking and baking, she taught us practical lessons, too. She had a routine that taught us organization and cooperation.

Siblings, Pets, and Other Disasters

Each Saturday morning, she awakened us early so we could clean the house. The three of us were to divide the chores and clean. When we were finished, the rest of the day was ours to do with as we pleased. We quickly learned that if we bickered, argued and wasted time, it took longer to get the jobs done and infringed on our leisure. If we cooperated, we had the majority of the day free. It was a lesson we learned well.

As a reward for a particularly peaceful, well-done job, we were sometimes allowed to go into town for a movie, if we had any money from our various jobs. One facet of that otherwise pleasant activity still grinds on me like a stone in my shoe. Even though I was younger, I was taller than my sister Linda. The ticket seller always insisted that I pay full price while Linda was admitted for the children's fee. Since we used our own hard earned money, I resented it bitterly.

In my life of mixed messages, there is one incident concerning my father that is as vivid to me now as it was the day it happened. It may have been the only time I every felt any compassion for him.

My grandparents had sold the island in Canada and now lived in Florida. When David was five, my mother flew down there with him to visit them over the Easter weekend. Despite his opinion of our friends at church, he had condescended to take us to church Easter morning. As we were dressing for church, the doorbell rang.

My father answered the door, and standing there was a florist delivery service. The young man had three live corsages for us. Mom had arranged their delivery before she left. My sisters and I were delirious. We hooted and jumped with joy.

When I looked at my father, expecting the usual dose of scorn and derision, I was surprised by what I saw. Tiny lines of pain etched the corners of his eyes. Wordlessly, he turned and went into the bedroom, softly closing the door behind him. I heard the door to his closet open and close. He didn't come out until time for church.

Later that day, my curiosity got the best of me, and I crept into his room as he dozed before the television set. Quietly, I opened the closet door. There, on the floor, were three plastic corsages. Sitting down on the floor by the closet, I wept silently. I wanted to put on those plastic flowers, tell my father that I loved him and wear that corsage with pride. But I didn't. It was too late, and I didn't have the courage to do it anyhow. Mostly, I feel sorry that my father died without ever learning how to express love.

That same summer I had a real vacation. Linda and I got to fly down to see my grandparents. We returned with backless sundresses adorned with colorful flowers and a pair of bright floppy earrings. We knew we were really cool. Both my father and my mother had other ideas. They teamed up to attack the way we looked. Words like trashy, smutty and tart brought the old double-edged sword down with a thwack! That seemed to be a trend. For every good thing in my life that made me feel like a real person, something negative evaporated the goodness with the speed of light.

Despite my poundage, with my height and bone structure an honest appraisal of the situation shows I was anything but fat. My thighs were a bit on the thick side but nowhere near fat. The taunts of "piano legs" still rang in my ears. I felt certain they were the size of oak trees. The monster had already altered my sense of perception.

This perception of being fat precipitated my first diet. Beverly and I decided to have a contest to see who could get down to one hundred twenty pounds first. Since I had no concept of dieting or nutrition, I simply skipped bread, potatoes, desserts and ate smaller portions. In an abortive way, I exercised with jumping jacks and fanny bumping sit-ups. At night, I ate a small portion of Rice Chexs very slowly. I won the contest with Beverly a close second.

Though the experience was unpleasant, I learned one thing. In my out of control life, I could control my weight. The seeds sown by the monster had sprouted, and a tiny plant was growing.

CHAPTER 5

School Days for Me and the Monster

School is basically a blur for me until the fourth grade. That winter, I had an upper respiratory infection and pneumonia that kept me out of school for four weeks. Despite mom's best home remedies for over two weeks, she was unable to cure the fevers, congestion and lethargy that daily embraced me. My parents were proud people. They would never do anything they couldn't pay for, and that included trips to the doctor with a sick child. When she finally scraped together enough money to pay for the visit to the doctor, I was extremely weak. He gave me a shot of penicillin, and in another ten days all symptoms were gone, and I headed back to class.

My teacher, Mrs. Overhaulser, became my heroine, my comforter and my inspiration. The diminutive, soft-spoken woman with the lustrous black hair spent countless extra hours bringing me up to speed and making up the lost material. Her patience, encouragement and the compliments she gave me resulted in the development of a smidgen of self-worth for the first time in my life. This gentle soul thought I was worth something, so I must be.

In Mrs. Overhaulser's classroom I picked up my first weapon to use in the battle with the demon. Later, it became a millstone. That weapon was control. This was a segment of my life I could control. If I worked hard and applied my God-given intellect, I could be the best student in my class. Here, it was relatively safe to compete and win. Here, I was someone. I belonged. Each morning when I collected my penny to buy milk at school, I was determined to be the best student I could possibly be. If I did, maybe I could stop being unwanted and become a real member of the Archer clan.

The weapon was effective. My parents took pride in my scholarly accomplishments. Compliments are hard for the anorexic personality to take, even when they are deserved. That trait was ingrained in me by fourth grade. Each compliment from my family was a barb, because even though I had earned it, I felt I didn't deserve it. Only in the classroom could I accept the accolades with any degree of self-satisfaction. Even though control proved to be a two edged sword, it didn't deter me from using control at the dinner table as a weapon, and over the years it nearly killed me.

Approaching high school, I had no social skills, no self-esteem and a generally unhealthy opinion of myself. Despite photographs that contradict my recollection, I felt that I was fat, unattractive and acne scarred. I weighed a whopping one hundred forty pounds. It was the most I have ever weighed in my life.

Though we were poor, we lived on the edge of an affluent area, and I attended Mentor High School. At that time, there were seventy to seventy-five kids per grade. It was a class-conscious atmosphere, and I was lower class by my own definition.

We rode the bus to school, while many of my classmates were driven there by their parents. A privileged few had their own cars. My lunch bags didn't help, either. We saved the paper lunch bags, using them over and over until the paper was so thin and shinny they looked like cloth. Eventually, they gave way with the embarrassing loss of a sandwich or apple on the floor of the bus. If bags were unavailable, mom wrapped our lunches in newspaper. I later learned that newsprint was sterile. Mom was simply ahead of her time, but it embarrassed me.

School Days for Me and the Monster

Had it not been for the gang of four, or the dork sisters as we sometime dubbed ourselves, high school would have been socially unbearable. Gale Holen and Judy Robinson joined Gayle Eisenburg and I to form a quartet of self-imposed outcasts.

We came from similar economic backgrounds. We never had dates, but had a whale of a good time with each other. We laughed, joked, talked on the phone for hours, painted our toenails and daydreamed together. When the effervescent Judy got the use of the family car, we all thought we had died and gone to heaven as we cruised the fifties drive-ins as if we were somebody.

The fact that no one ever asked me for a date in high school merely confirmed my feeling of worthlessness. I retreated from the usual teenage social scene with a pen pal named Fritz who lived in Norway. Although our correspondence was never romantic, I still daydreamed about him. But, my old friend, the two-edged sword wouldn't leave me to my fantasy.

Fritz came to the United States on vacation and actually came to my home to see me. He was a pleasant, handsome young man with impeccable manners, and we had as peaceful a dinner as a family that I could remember. Unfortunately, at the sight of Fritz, I came apart at the seams. Seeing Fritz and my father at the same table, all sorts of wild thoughts flashed through my head. Unable to interact in a reasonable way with him, I drew into a shell and became nearly mute. When Fritz left that night, I never saw or heard from him again. It remains a sad memory for me.

My major social outing in high school involved my friends and my sister, Linda. The Girl's Athletic Association at our school sponsored a formal dance, and since it was a girl-ask- boy affair, we decided to be bold and ask boys from our MYF group to go with us.

We had a great time getting ready for the big night with strapless gowns, corsages and new hairstyles. After getting our pictures taken, we went to the dance. Since the boys weren't from our school, they didn't know anybody. They had less social skills than we did and couldn't dance.

Although we laughed and did the silly things teenagers do, the night wasn't ideal. But, it was the best night out the misfits could muster.

One other social encounter is worthy of mention. When I was sixteen, a friend of one of my neighbors spied me sunbathing one day. He stopped over and asked me to go to a movie. He was twenty-five and not a bad looking chap. Despite the age difference, my parents allowed me to go out with him, mostly because he was a friend of our neighbors.

The evening began innocently enough with a trip to the theater. I have no idea what the movie was about, but after half-an-hour, he decided the movie wasn't to his liking, and we left the theater. Suggesting we go for a walk, he led me eventually to a sheltered spot where he kissed me.

Flattered by the attention of an "older man", I kissed him back. Immediately his hands started to move, and in thirty seconds the encounter turned into either a major league grope or a class one assault, I could never quite determine which.

Breaking the hold, I wiggled away and demanded that he take me home at once. He did, and fortunately, I never heard from him again, directly. Indirectly, I did. He took his revenge for the slight to his manhood.

Roughly a week later, my father stormed into the house hurling invectives at me.

"So, you're a hot potato! Is that right? The boys all tell me you're a hot potato! Are you?" he screamed, his face so red I was sure he would have a stroke!

In the early fifties, a hot potato was the equivalent of a slut. Since I had done nothing wrong, the insult infuriated me even more. Coming from my father, it was even worse. Was he so angry because he thought I might be giving someone else what I had refused him? I can't be sure, but I'm convinced that had to be part of it. The incident ignited one more donnybrook that my poor brother never understood.

God had given me a brain and the ability to use it. Study was an excuse to stay in my room and out of the line of fire. I became one of the best students in my high school. But, the two edged sword cut my joy into a dichotomy.

I can never remember being rewarded for good grades or academic accomplishments. There was only the criticism and punishment if I didn't get an A in every subject. When I got a B, you'd have thought I failed the course. Fortunately, the B's didn't come often.

On the other hand, Linda was rewarded with precious money for making a B in a subject. Each time it happened, it infuriated me and sent me scowling for the refuge of my room to rail at the injustice of it. I realize now that Linda had more difficulty in school than I did, and it was my parent's way of trying to help and encourage her. I blamed Linda for it at the time, believing she was getting special attention. If my parents had possessed more communications skills, a few words to me would have helped me to understand and perhaps avoid my resentment. Unfortunately, they didn't have them.

Dave also rained on my academic parade. Each time he entered a new class, he was greeted with, "Oh, you're Pat's brother." Dave, who has always had difficulty accepting responsibility for his own actions or shortcomings, used me as the excuse for his poor academic record.

"After they found out I was your brother, I never had a chance," he hurled at me later in life.

When he made the accusation, I was ensconced in the victim roll and accepted it as fact. Immediately, I entered the acceptance mode and agreed that it was my fault and offering profuse apologies. Since I'm no longer a victim, I realize that it wasn't my fault. I worked hard and applied myself, striving to be the best I could be. If that set a high standard, I won't apologize.

Academic success was my way of proving self worth when I had very little. It proved to me that I could succeed in the world when my home life discouraged me from believing that I could. Since I was an acne scarred, fat body that no one could really love, including my family, I would have to be able to support myself. That became the focus and driving force of my high school years.

Discovering the Monster Within

Approaching graduation, the tension in our house increased geometrically, or at least my perception of it did. Many teens see high school graduation as a watershed in their lives for a number of reasons. I had only one. After graduation, I would be free to pursue my dream of being a nurse. And, I could leave the house of discord forever.

In May of 1958 I celebrated my eighteenth birthday. September of that year, I began the pursuit of my dream to become a nurse. In my conscious mind, I had the double goal of helping people and proving my father wrong about my ability. And, in my subconscious mind, I had a desperate need to control my life.

Such feelings are not unusual for the anorexic. Many of us are enablers, faithful handmaidens or obedient servants. Like the eldest child, we strive to please in the hope that it will gain us love and acceptance. Simultaneously, we battle to control lives that our subconscious perceives to be careening down the highway of life like an out of control racecar. As a nurse, I could control my environment, at least at work.

With my usual trepidation concerning new things, I packed my meager belongings, and my folks drove me to the dormitory at The Cleveland Metropolitan Hospital's School of Nursing. Though we lived in the dorm at Metro, we were bused to the Francis Payne Bolton Nursing School at Case Western Reserve University for basic science classes such as chemistry, microbiology and anatomy. I loved it there because Wade Park was nearby, and it was safe to wander there at lunchtime on sunny days. How time has changed that. It isn't safe anymore.

As my folks drove away, I was torn by the dual emotions of excited anticipation and sheer terror. Shy and backward, lacking all but the most rudimentary social skills, I was certain the other girls (we had no men in our class), wouldn't accept me. What does that say about my self worth? Deciding my only option was to be the best student I could be, I approached my training days with the mindset of a novice headed for the convent.

We had single rooms as freshman. Only the top students in the class, determined by competitive exams at the end of the freshman year, were allowed to have roommates. It marked the first time in my entire life that I had a room of my own. It was a God send, because with everything else chipping away at what little self-confidence I had, I'm not sure I would have handled a roommate very well. Despite having shared a room my whole life with a sister, my own dread of social interaction petrified me. I felt ill equipped to handle daily conversation with a perfect stranger.

As we gathered for our group orientation meeting, I surveyed the eager faces in the room, and it made me feel worse. They were cheerful, happy, enthusiastic and bantered with each other as if they were life-long friends. I sat quietly by myself feeling totally inept.

I realize now, that it was my perception of me, and not what the other girls saw. But, it was the only way I knew how to interpret things then. Anorexics have both a problem with input and output. We learn, very early in life, to warp what is said to us and what was meant by it into something entirely different than the speaker intended. Relearning these skills becomes a paramount hurdle in therapy.

Rooms were assigned alphabetically. My room was at the head of one of the four sides of a quadrangle surrounding a patio garden that would be my world for the next three years. There was a telephone at each of the four corners of the quadrangle. I thought our phone at home got congested with three girls and one phone. Four phones and so many young women redefined chaos.

I used one of those phones to call home after my first few days at school. Just like Bible camp, I was homesick. Things were too quiet and peaceful in the dorm. Part of me still longed for the confusion and criticism of the Archer house.

My father answered the phone. I asked if I could come home for the weekend, and he told me no. I wanted to get away to school, so I could just stay there. I was crushed, but in time I got over it and settled into my new surroundings.

My social ineptness made it hard for the other girls to get to know me. I usually responded with grunts and monosyllables, discouraging normal conversations. As I observed my classmates in action, I crawled further into my shell. I tried to make myself invisible.

Many of the girls came from bigger, ritzier high schools than I did. High school was easy for me. I learned a great deal of technical information, but I was ignorant concerning literature, history or music. When the other girls talked about it, I felt like a real bimbo.

It would be easy to blame my high school for my shoddy liberal arts background. In truth, my high school did offer liberal arts courses, but I wasn't interested in them. They served no purpose in preparing me for nurses training. In addition, I had no exposure to such things at home. At home, if it wasn't sports, or perhaps Lawrence Welk, my father could have cared less, and my mother was too tired for culture.

My hair proved to be the prow of the icebreaker that parted the frozen sea separating me from my classmates. Since I was an Archer and Sue was a Burden, we lived on the same hall. She told me that the rest of the class had questions about my hair. Was the color natural? What did I put on it? It was so light and blond, they all wondered. I told her it was natural, and we began to talk about that and other things. I had made my first friend. Forty years later, Sue Burden Deville and I are still friends.

Later, I found that some of the girls had taken turns following me to the shower room to see what I put on my hair. They thought I had lied to Sue about my hair being natural. It disturbed me at the time. I couldn't imagine why they would think I'd lie about something as trivial as that. Being a social misfit had the advantage of depriving me of the guile many young girls develop as a defense mechanism. Blond hair never bothered me. I even enjoy blond jokes. Well, most of them anyhow.

A second person who helped me adjust was Jeanette "Suzie" Schzycheck. Each freshman was assigned an advisor to help them handle the roller coaster ride of that first year in training. We called them big sisters. Suzie was mine, and I couldn't have had a better one.

School Days for Me and the Monster

Suzie now has six children and still works full time nightshift. She's a living inspiration to those women who want a family and a career. She has successfully juggled both and is the perfect rebuttal to my father's interpretation of the role of women in our society.

As nursing students, we had free medical care. One of the first things they did was to give us a complete physical examination. My acne didn't escape their attention.

They began with the usual treatment of antibiotics and Physohex scrubs. When that proved ineffective, they incised and drained the larger pockets. Then, they fed the young monster. They placed me on a strict, low fat diet that was standard therapy for acne sufferers in the fifties.

The diet consisted of dry steaks, chops, or chicken, no salad dressing and no fat whatsoever. It gave me something in my life to control, and control it I did. The diet became my religion. I restricted not only fat but also anything that even resembled it. When I came back from my first extended break over Thanksgiving, I had gained three pounds. I was already weighing myself frequently. The monster told me I should watch my weight very carefully.

Looking into the mirror, I heard my father's voice inside my head. "Bustle Butt, Bustle Butt." My hips didn't need desserts. Neither did my face. I'll remove those to the diet along with most starches. The monster inside chuckled.

This new decision proved a boon for my classmates and increased my popularity.

Suddenly people battled to sit with me at mealtime. I felt honored to have so much attention, until I found that they were only interested in the dessert I refused to touch.

I made another important discovery that first year in nurses training. I am a visual learner, and because high school had been so easy for me, I really didn't know how to study. When we studied physiology and talked about things like adduction and abduction, the way joints move, I wiggled around contorting my body in an attempt to visualize

79

the movements. Although my classmates though I was a bit strange, it worked, until classes like pharmacy, and chemistry came along.

Fortunately, Sue Burden came to my rescue. Sue is very bright and a great teacher. Energetic, bubbly, loving and supportive, Sue's room resembled Auntie Em's place when Dorothy returned from Oz. Despite the clutter and disorganization, Sue's mind was a steel trap when it came to information. She is a brilliant woman whose life is a model of success, and I have always been proud of her accomplishments. Today, Sue is a professor at Baldwin Wallace College.

She took me under her wing and made me feel special. Using her talent for teaching, she showed me how to organize, helped me with note taking and all the goofy little drawings that are so important to the understanding of medical subjects. Sue gave me hints on what to focus on, how to remember the important things and not be so concerned with every little detail. Without her help, I never would have made it through nurses training.

The tension of that first year exacerbated my sleepwalking tendencies. Several times that year, I somnambulated my way around the old quadrangle. My first nocturnal romp still provides me with a chuckle. I woke up in the middle of one of our four hallways. I had no idea which hallway it was. Fortunately, the four phones had different progressive numbers. Hustling to the phone, I looked at the number. My phone was two numbers higher than the one I was holding. Realizing I was on the opposite corner of the quad, I sheepishly made my way back to my room.

Another interesting result of the first year pressure was the cessation of my menstrual periods. Had I been sexually active then, it would have been a source of great concern. Had I still been my father's victim, I honestly believe I might have become suicidal. Since the only pregnancy I was likely to be party to at this juncture in my life would have required Immaculate Conception, I welcomed the state of affairs as one inconvenience I wouldn't have to bother with.

School Days for Me and the Monster

Reflecting on the situation, cessation of menstrual periods is a sign of anorexia as well. I wonder how much my nearly anorexic diet during training exacerbated the amenorrhea.

Although there was no dating during the first year of training, (try that on today's modern women,) we did attend socials at some of the Case Western fraternity houses. With my limited social background I was shocked at what went on there.

We went as a group to the I Grabba Thigh Fraternity house and found it chock full of aggressive young men whose testosterone levels dwarfed their IQs. Music throbbed through the dimly lit structure, base notes hammering hard enough to set my fillings on edge. A bathtub filled with ice held enough bottles of beer to supply a military regiment on a forty-eight hour pass. The bottles quickly became a mountain of empties in the corner as the young men ferried back and forth to the tub like worker bees feeding the queen.

The social portion of the party was relegated to lightning negotiating sessions. A man would introduce himself, while mentally undressing me. A few polite questions, whose answers didn't seem to concern him in the least, preceded his invitation to dance. After a dance floor grope, the invitation to a more intimate session followed while he was still trying to recall my name. When I refused, he disappeared like Casper the Friendly Ghost when the sun comes up. For those of us who chose to remain grope-less, the evening turned into a boring spectacle of drunkenness that was an all too familiar to me. I had seen my father like this all too often.

To be fair, I gave it one more chance. After the second social proved to be a carbon copy of the first, I didn't attend any more fraternity parties.

The other social event I attended I lovingly recall as hen parties. A half dozen girls would bop off to the pizza parlor after a hard night of hitting the books. My acne diet gave me the perfect excuse to enjoy the party but forgo the pizza. I had a cola, diet of course.

Discovering the Monster Within

Pizza was never my forte. I don't suppose I've had more than half a dozen slices of pizza in my life. When I was tempted, which was rare, I found that by going immediately to the bathroom and using my well-honed skills at visualization, I could set the stage for a first class purge. I never had to resort to the finger down the throat trick. A few calculated strokes on the outside of my throat and the tasty morsels came up without a hitch. Every time I did, the monster chuckled. I eased into the behavior as naturally as taking a drink of water. This also places Pizza on my list of foods that will be hard to incorporate into my recovering diet.

Although I could justify not eating just about anything, I continued to eat those items I was allowed to eat. I was not yet totally anorexic. I like to think of myself during this period as a Situational Bulimic. My weight remained in the one hundred thirty pound range. Nearing the end of that first year, I started to feel fat again. I'm not sure what the trigger was, but I began to worry about my weight constantly. Multiple, daily trips to the scales insinuated their way into my routine, and the monster laughed.

When I felt stressed, particularly near test time, I would eat half a bag of potato chips or a whole bar of candy. Consumed by guilt, I performed my magic trick, and the offending calories vanished into the toilet bowl. I could do that as often as I wanted too and not gain an ounce. And, the monster roared with glee.

As I try to recall the severity of the disorder in those early years, I now realize it was worse than I remember. Although we had a continuous three years of training, we did get some weekends off and occasionally a longer break with a holiday. Nothing had changed at the Archer house, so when I came home, I worked as much as I could baby sitting. I needed the money, and everyone liked a future nurse looking after little Johnnie or Janie.

Occasionally, I ate junk food with my clients, which I immediately brought back up in the usual fashion. When I decided to splurge, I ate huge quantities of junk. As any good bulimic will tell you, the more you eat, the easier it is to bring it back up. I wasn't yet to the point of stuffing myself with ridiculous amounts of food and purging. Still, this was good training.

I didn't purge much at home, but something about my behavior obviously made my mother suspicious, because she questioned me about it. Of course I denied everything. If my mother was so observant about my eating, it makes me wonder how much she knew about other things.

On one of my sojourns home, my sister, Beverly, bought me a two-piece brown dress that I remember with affection to this day. I weighed one hundred twenty-eight pounds the day she gave it to me, and I immediately decided that was too much. The dress would be much more attractive if I weighed a couple of pounds less. I was in control of my weight now, and it would be no problem. And, the monster danced with glee.

At the end of the first academic year, we had a competitive examination. Sue Burden and I passed and became roommates. At last, I felt like I belonged. I really knew I could make it through nurse's training. I was in control of my life, and the monster and I loved that.

During the second year we started such daunting clinical services as obstetrics and gynecology, surgery, medicine and pediatrics, but I was ready. I was determined to be perfect, not only because I wanted to for myself, but to prove my father wrong about me.

Of all the rotations, medicine was the favorite. It provided me with an intellectual boost that still causes me to blush when I recount it. One task on medicine was to choose a patient and do an in-depth nursing care assessment. Details concerning the patient, his religion, family, occupation and a host of other facts were obtained as well as a comprehensive review of the patient's medical problem. All these things are then correlated and compiled in a lengthy report relating all the places in the patient's life where nursing intervention might be helpful. When our instructor, Mrs. Welsh, returned my paper, it had an A on the top and a single word, perfect.

Discovering the Monster Within

Later, Mrs. Welsh came to me privately and asked if she might use my case report as the example of how it should be done in her future classes.

With a blush like a blooming rose I stammered, "Of course you can."

Later some of the underclassmen stopped me in the hallway to commend my accomplishment. If it hadn't been against school rules, my pride filled chest might have popped the buttons off my stiffly starched uniform endangering passers by with flying debris.

My social life for most of the next two years was twofold. Most enjoyable were the weekends with Sue Burden. Her mother was a gem and one of the most personable people I've ever met. Sue had two siblings, an older sister, Sandy, and a younger brother, Dick. They were both as bright as Sue, and to watch them together and join in the repartee was wonderful.

They were a low income, middle class working family, and I felt truly at home with them. Unfortunately, there was something else there that made me feel at home. Sue's father was an alcoholic, too, though he lacked the venom mine possessed. A quiet, distant person, when he arrived home from work, he poured a beer, added a shot of whiskey and drank it. The ritual was repeated over and over until he fell asleep. His monster killed him at an early age.

They lived in an old house in Cleveland, and it reminded me so much of my own home. Despite her father's problem, Sue's house was filled with love and kindness and a unity that mine sorely lacked. When I was there, I could pretend I was part of that family rather than my own.

Food was always an integral part of these visits. Sue's mom was the perfect hostess, and she fed us as if she feared they didn't feed us at the dorm. My skills at regurgitation became a science on those weekends. I also learned to do it so my friends wouldn't notice. My monster gave me an A on that project.

My second outlet was Sunday visits to my parent's friends Eva and Donald's home for dinner. They were friends of my parents, and when

I didn't go home for the weekend, I had a standing invitation to their home for dinner.

Dinner there was an event. Plates were piled high with food in some of the largest servings I have ever seen before or since. Eva and Donald tried hard to make me feel at home. Both of them were obese and Donald died young. I remember how they complained that I always ate like a bird.

No! I did not eat like a bird! Birds are marvels of God's creation with metabolic rates that make the most hyperactive human pale by comparison. Birds are ravenous eaters, some species consuming more food than their body weight daily. When you live with a monster, you learn a lot about eating habits.

A sin I once committed on those visits was indulging in cinnamon toast slathered with butter. Their son, Butch, loved that in the evening. I still feel guilty about it, especially since I didn't always bring it back up. I managed to get rid of most of the huge portions they fed me. I hadn't yet refined the fine art of food juggling and avoidance, so I relied on bulimic behavior to preserve my shrinking waistline.

They had a daughter, too. Annie was younger than Butch, and she really didn't stand a chance. From a young age, her father force-fed her, producing an obese child that has had to fight her weight her entire life.

As I observed their overeating, I became aware of something more terrifying. I was mortally afraid of becoming fatter. I saw myself through the eyes of my parents. I already felt fat. I never could see myself as I really was, another unfortunate circumstance for anorexics. I knew that one more serving of mashed potatoes, one more spoonful of custard would push me over the top, and I would make the quantum leap from fat to morbidly obese in a heartbeat. It caused me to quake with fear and check the scales repeatedly, and I began to practice dietary restriction. Unfortunately, I thought it was the healthy thing to do. My monster told me it was. My monster would never lie to me.

Discovering the Monster Within

As I entered the clinical services, there seemed to be an overwhelming amount of material to learn. In my quest for perfection, I studied even harder than before. It proved a fertile field for my eating disorder.

When tension levels were particularly high, it was not unusual for me to eat an entire box of ginger snaps and then vomit them up a few minutes after the last one went down. My favorite snack foods included Life Savers and those delicious little caramel candies filled with white cream. I learned to make a Life Saver last an hour and a caramel cream three hours. Of course even those had to come back up in the end. I was practicing for my anorexic restriction phase when I would be able to make a lettuce leaf last through a seven-course meal.

Thinking back, I'm not sure if I've ever truly enjoyed food. Though it's hard for me to image now, fried chicken, mashed potatoes, corn on the cob, and turkey with that golden brown skin still intact were my favorites along with my mom's baked goods. Thanks to ED, I haven't tasted those things for years. Now that I must eat healthier foods in an attempt to shore up the damage I have done to myself, I will likely never enjoy those foods again. I do eat corn now, but always plain, and chicken is never fried. The combination of my self-image, fueled by parental criticism and negativity and the turmoil at the table have robbed me of the pleasures of mealtime.

To me a pound overweight was the same as fifty pounds over. My appearance was always unacceptable to me since I allowed my self- image to be formulated by my parents. As far as I was concerned, obesity was the worst sin a woman could ever commit. I labeled myself, and it became ingrained into my personality. Other people, regardless of their size were acceptable to society, but not me. I was too fat. Only now do I understand how that lie contaminated my life.

My relationship with my classmates improved over the next two years. They elected me president of our senior class, so I know that's true. Most of the tension and pressure I felt was self- imposed. I convinced myself that the reason for their largess was that they respected my dedication and work ethic. Right? Wrong? That may have been part of it, but I must have been a likeable *person,* too.

Self-worth and identity are the monster's major weapons. I had a secure foundation of neither. Now, I know I am a real person. I am likeable for whom I am. My classmates accepted my idiosyncrasies, just as I accepted theirs. I don't know why it's so hard for us with the monster to understand that. But, since I didn't like myself much back then, it took me nearly a lifetime to learn that simple fact.

A fond recollection of the training years was our choir. I love to sing, despite the fact that I can't carry a tune in a bucket. If someone who *can* carry a tune is next to me, I can find the notes and do an acceptable job. The girls knew how much I liked to sing, so they put me between two of the best voices in the choir, and I sang my little heart out. I have never learned the tune thing, so I confine most of my vocal renditions to the shower where the sound of running water evens things out.

Dating was allowed over the final two years, but in general it's not a pleasant memory for me. There were other social events that were suspiciously like fraternity parties. The guy would come over and put his arm on the back of my chair. Then he recited the story of his usually disastrous life. Searching for acceptance, he was certain I was his salvation. One chap creatively assured me that as the result of a horrible accident, he was permanently sterile, thus safe to be with.

Usually, I left these parties with some of the other girls. One night, I made the mistake of accepting a ride to the dorm from a young man. Over my protest, instead of taking me home, he drove to his apartment. When I refused to go inside, he began a direct frontal assault that was difficult to repulse. In the end, he ejaculated all over my new pink dress! That soured me on dating for months.

I did meet one young man who behaved with more alacrity. He had more patience than the rest. He was the closest thing to a real boyfriend I had ever had. We dated several times. Slowly, he became bolder. When he realized I wasn't going to give him what he was after, he dropped me like a bad habit. I kind of liked him, and it was another hammer blow to my fragile ego.

Although I felt sure I had a healthy sexual attitude, I realize that I didn't. What I interpreted as Neanderthal behavior was really standard operating procedure for young men who were as nervous and insecure as I was as they attempted the transformation from teenager to manhood. Most of my classmates handled it far better than I did, and most of them survived with their virginities intact. Considering my family history, I should have realized that my criticism was unduly caustic. Still, that's how I felt then.

I tried to convince myself that I wasn't interested in dating or sex. It was another carefully constructed defense. If I wasn't dating, I wouldn't put myself in a position to be threatened with the possibility of a sexual encounter. Without realizing it, when faced with a man's aggressive sexual behavior, I was subconsciously back in my bedroom at home warding off the unwanted advances of my father.

One of the final portions of our training included a rotation on obstetrics and gynecology. A two-week stint in the outpatient clinic was part of the training. The hospital was enormous, and the cavernous clinic held rows of benches filled with the poor and indigent souls of Cuyahoga County who couldn't find or afford health care anywhere else.

The clinic was a real eye-opener for me. One of my first cases was a fourteen-year-old girl in her first trimester of pregnancy. The unfortunate child had no idea that she was pregnant and was completely clueless as to how pregnancies occurred. Street wise beyond here years, she was already an expert in the technical aspects of sex but lacked even rudimentary knowledge of its consequences.

A wild woman managed the clinic and supervised the students. Bright, energetic and efficient, she ran the show like the top drill sergeant in a boot camp. When she moved, things got done. Her name was Kathleen Elizabeth Burkley, and she became my instant heroine. I wanted to be a nurse exactly like her, and I worked my tail off in that clinic.

My attitude and work ethic caught her eye, and she took me under her wing. One afternoon over a cup of coffee in the lounge, she asked me if I was dating anyone.

"No, not really," I said.

Hesitantly, she continued. "I have a son named, Art. He's not dating anyone either. Do you think you might like to go out with him?"

"Sure," I replied with more enthusiasm than I felt.

It wasn't an unusual request from a senior nurse. If they had a son who wasn't the best material, was shy, withdrawn, or lacked the social skills to fend for himself, their mothers played matchmaker with eligible nursing students. I was seldom the target of such a request, but this time, out of respect for Kathleen, I accepted. Besides, I was tired of watching all the other girls go out while I sat at home in the dorm.

Two nights later, one of the corner gang phones rang, and someone shouted, "Pat!"

Pat Klemencic answered the summons, and since I seldom got any outside calls, I thought nothing more of it. About an hour later, Pat came sheepishly into my room.

"Are you working obstetrical clinic now?" she asked.

"Yes. It's my second week. Why?" I replied.

"I think I just accepted a date from the guy you were supposed to go out with. He's Mrs. Burkley's son, Art," she said blushing with embarrassment.

Laughing, I said, "Don't sweat it. That's fine by me. I like Mrs. Burkley and didn't want to say no. You know how I am about blind dates. Go have a ball. I'm not mad. Actually, you did me a favor."

With a sigh of relief, she said, "Thanks Pat."

"But," I added in my best schoolteacher voice, "I want a full report on my desk in the morning."

I didn't have to wait until morning. Around midnight she came back to my room.

"He' really a very nice guy," Pat began. "He took me to a hockey game. Afterwards, we went for a bite to eat, and he brought me straight home. He's quiet and polite to a fault. I explained the mix-up to him, and he took it pretty well. He's going to call you. I think that's best. He's really not my type. You can have him," she said, and went back to her room chuckling to herself.

I sat there thinking about what she had just said. I wasn't sure if I was pleased, insulted or angry. She didn't want him so I could have him. Did I want her leftovers? What exactly was my type, and what did she mean by that? Since I didn't have time to worry about it right then, I went back to my work with a shrug, and put the incident out of my mind.

Two days later, a soft spoken, polite young man called me on the phone and asked me to go out with him. I accepted his invitation, and it changed my life forever.

CHAPTER 6

The Love of My Life

There are truly three parts to a person's nuclear family. The Archer family fulfilled the role as my family of origin. The family I ultimately married into was my husband's family of origin. Together my husband and I formed a new nuclear family, bringing with us the baggage of each of our families of origin. For anorexics, these complex human interactions play an important role in the development, enablement and progression of the disease as well as its cure. At times, the best of intentions by the family has disastrous results for the anorexic individual. Unintentionally, a families concern and treatment of the anorexic enables the monster and allows it to roam unchallenged. At one time or another, all these things were in play with me.

Because these things are so important in the life of an anorexic, I want to devote an entire chapter to my husband, Arthur Burkley, because not only is he the love of my life, and the only man I have ever loved, but also he saved my life. Like any relationship spanning more than four decades, it has had its share of rocky spots. At times, our boat seemed about to dash on those rocks. But, one thing remains crystal clear. Without the constant support and unselfish love given to me by my husband, I wouldn't be alive to recount this narrative.

Discovering the Monster Within

By today's standards, my first date with my future mate was extraordinarily tame. It was, and I loved it. But, things were different in the fifties.

After straightening out which Pat had been called for a date, I accepted Art's invitation. The next night, nervous as a cat in a dog pound, I took a deep breath and walked from my room to the reception area where Prince Charming awaited.

When I first saw him, he was standing there with his dark top coat open, a cigarette rakishly held, European style, deep between his fingers where they joined his hand. He was beautiful. And, he was too small!

I'm five feet seven with a solid bone structure. At least it was solid before ED showed me how to weaken it. If not for my monster, I could easily carry one hundred thirty pounds. When I first met Art, I weighed one thirteen. I never saw myself as thin.

Although Art is taller than I am, he has a lithe frame, and even today possesses a boyish look that is the envy of our friends and makes him appear ten years younger than he is. As I looked at him standing there in the lounge, I knew this was never going to work. I was a moose, and he was a pony. I decided to make the best of things for this one evening.

An immediate difference between Art and the other men I had dated was his politeness. I had never known anyone who opened doors for me, stayed on his side of the car, and acted as if he truly respected me. ED reminded me that I didn't deserve such treatment. Unfortunately, I agreed.

We went to a Cleveland Baron's hockey game at the old arena on Euclid and Thirtieth Street. The entire experience was new to me. Art patiently tried to explain the rules, and although I strove to develop a feel for the contest, I never became a true hockey fan.

During one rapid exchange, the puck ricocheted off the glass and arched into the stands. Art outwrestled several other men who frantically clawed the air as if the rubber disk were made of gold. Art was elated when he caught the puck, and he proudly presented it to me. Thanking him, I tucked his treasure into my purse.

The Love of My Life

Not being a hockey aficionado, I pondered what I was going to do with this dumb piece of round rubber. Eventually, I gave it to my dog Duke, who became very fond of it. Later, when Art came to meet my folks, he found Duke gnawing on his hard earned prize. I'm sure Art thought I would cherish it forever. I guess I'm not the sentimental type.

After the game, we went to Kenny Kings for cheeseburgers and coffee. Mostly we talked. We talked for hours. We talked on all our dates about everything and anything. Art jokingly says that we talked so much when we were dating that he had nothing left to say after we got married.

We lost track of time, and it was late when we got back to the dorm that night. Pat Klemencic was waiting for me, and she was full of questions.

"Where have you been? What were you doing? "

I flashed my best Mona Lisa smile and left the answers to her fertile imagination. I didn't tell her that he was so polite he didn't even try to kiss me good night. It was easier to ignore her than it was ED. I did as my monster told me, but it was too late. The offending cheeseburger had already infiltrated my system. It was at times like these that I first began to feel small ripples of panic because of the absorbed calories. I shuddered to think of what it would do to my waistline.

That first date began our whirlwind courtship. It was a fairy tail for me. Art took me to Severance Hall to see the Cleveland Symphony Orchestra perform. Art's parents had been there for the inaugural performance in the hall in nineteen thirty-one. I had never been inside the building, and I thought it was wonderful.

My favorites were the Orchestra's summer concerts at the old Convention Center Concert Hall. They were informal events where the audience was seated at round tables. Food and drinks were for sale. They were elegantly informal, and I loved them, the drinks not the food.

We visited the Drury Theater for plays and the Carrousel Theater for outdoor musicals. On other occasions we went to the Columbia Ball

Room to dance to the forties sound of a live big band. For once, I was grateful for the dance lessons after the A.A. meetings. In Art's arms, I felt none of the terror I did when I danced with my father.

On our second date, we saw a movie called *Carry On Nurse*. It contained risqué scenes that made me squirm, but Art took them good naturedly. I was unsure how I would handle any sexual situation, and that bothered me more than what was happening on the screen.

We took long walks in neighborhood parks and parked near the Cleveland Hopkins Airport to watch the planes come in. At least I think there were planes there, or maybe submarines. Never did I feel threatened by anything we did.

While I could scarcely believe my good fortune, the old sword of dichotomy took a swipe at me again. Art was handsome, charming, polite, comfortable to be with, the impeccable gentleman, and most of all, safe! He made no demands on me and seemed to truly enjoy being with me. My jury still deliberated about his size.

On the other hand, my monster played on my insecurity with such questions as, "What does he see in you? Are you sure you're worth it? What's he going to say when he finds out about your old man? Goodbye, Prince Charming. You're not good enough for him and he knows it. You're from the wrong side of the tracks. Besides, you're fat and acne scarred."

I tried to convince myself that I wasn't ready for a full time relationship like this. I had special feelings for Art, but denied that I might love him. Retrospectively, it was a defense mechanism to protect me from being hurt again. Almost every man I ever knew had let me down, and eventually this one would, too. It was my zero self worth at work again. Interestingly, it was food that told me how special he was.

Nearly every time we went out, we grabbed a bite to eat, either before or after the main event of the evening. Our favorite place was Bearden's, a hamburger joint owned by Gene Bearden, the Cleveland Indian's shortstop at the time. The specialty of the house was a peanut burger. They were hamburgers slathered with peanut butter and sweet relish. As gross as it sounds, we both loved them.

As soon as I wiped the grease from my chin from the last bite, ED was in my face. "Get rid of it! Get rid of it!" he demanded. But, I felt so good when I was with Art that I told ED to stuff it! I refused to do my magic trick.

Apparently, I impressed my future mother in law more than I realized. Years later, I discovered that shortly after I began to date Art, she zeroed in on me as a future member of the family. Kathleen ran the family the same way she ran the clinic. She was a possessive, controlling woman who manipulated others like marionettes on a string through the strength of her personality. I was not fully aware of the scope of her influence until much later in our relationship, when it became more fuel for the monster's pyre.

As a result of our long walks and talks, I learned a great deal about Art's family and their values. Since my family never had much money, I had learned to live without it. Art's family placed a great deal of emphasis on the accumulation of wealth, and had no sympathy for the slackers of the world. I wasn't sure if I could identify with that philosophy. They also had little tolerance for the slow-witted or fat people. I was certain I could handle those two. I wasn't slow-witted, and I'd *never* be fat. I'd rather die than be fat. I knew that for certain now.

Since I now knew Art's philosophy of life, I tried to define what mine was. After much deliberation, I came to the unsettling conclusion that I didn't have a philosophy of life! I didn't want to be the way my parents were, and I wasn't sure I could be like Art's folks. With the exception of my decision to attend nursing school, I had spent my whole life trying to be what someone else wanted me to be. I viewed myself through other people's eyes. I had no idea who I was or what I believed in. Could I see myself through Kathleen's eyes and be that person?

The first time we went to Art's home, I was overwhelmed. It was Sunday afternoon, and Kathleen was dressed as if she were going to church. Art's dad, Arthur W. Burkley, was dressed in a white shirt, tie and jacket. Kathleen served cake and coffee on a table that was as impeccable as the manners they used. It was like something from an Ozzie and Harriet show, and as far from my hectic family life as New York is from Hong Kong. I left that day convinced that I would never live up to their rigorous standards.

When I saw Art's dad the second time, the Ozzie Nelson image vanished in an instant. The two Burkley men were renovating an old house, and Art took me there to view their handiwork. It was a hot day, and when we arrived, Art senior was at the top of a stepladder perspiring like a waterfall. To keep the sweat out of his eyes, he had fashioned a headband from a Kotex pad. As I struggled to keep from rolling on the floor with laughter, I realize Dad Burkley was an O. K. guy, and I had nothing to fear from him.

Then, the two edged sword sliced the air like Poe's blade from the Pit. Whatever work Art's dad was doing, and I don't remember what it was, didn't suit the younger Burkley, and my Prince Charming threw the classic hissie-fit. Taking off his watch, he flung it across the room, where it slammed into the wall. The pedestal I had placed Art on collapsed with a crash. Strangely, the ugly behavior caused me to relax. Until now, Art had been nothing short of perfect. That act made him imperfect, like me, and I could handle imperfection. I never considered his temper could be a problem. Strange how ones sees what they want to see isn't it?

Eventually, Art had to meet my parents, and the thought of that filled me with anxiety. His first impression of my mother was straight from a slap sick comedy routine. When we arrived at the Johnny Cake house, mom was in the yard with our dog Duke. No big deal. Right? Wrong!

Duke was a peculiar animal who thought he was a she and squatted to urinate like a female dog. Since Duke's anatomy was ill suited for such behavior, he routinely urinated on his own chin whiskers. If that wasn't disgusting enough, he also liked to lick your cheek.

Mom had begun a campaign to teach Duke how to urinate the proper way for a male dog. When her future son-in-law came to meet her, my mother was in the yard holding up Duke's back leg while he urinated in a vain attempt to teach an old dog a new trick. Later, when Duke bounded into the room with Art's prize puck in his teeth, Art was crushed. I don't think he ever liked Duke all that much.

Duke went out of his way to torment the Burkley boys. Mom kept Duke hooked by a chain on a run in the back yard. Later on, Art's brother, Lew, came to visit and was enjoying one of mom's doughnuts when Duke wrapped the chain around Lew's leg. Turning, Duke dashed for the doghouse, donut in mouth, nearly taking Lew's leg with him.

Mom fell immediately in love with Art, and my father disliked him with equal rapidity. Art had an education. It thrilled my mother and infuriated my father. Art's interests, personality and values were the opposite of my father's. Though they were opposite of my mother's too, she realized how special Art was and loved him at once.

Just as I wish my brother, Dave, could have known the mother of my earlier years, I wish Art could have, too. I know Art liked her, but I doubt he ever truly loved her. She was a crusty Gal who loved us fiercely but had a hard time showing it. She was worn out by the time he met her, but he admits she was one of the hardest working people he has ever met. She had a good heart and meant well, but while my father was alive, she was gnarly and defensive. After he died, and she had to support herself, she mellowed some, but the bitterness never completely disappeared.

My father revealed his dry drunk personality that first day with Art, setting the tone for an antagonistic relationship between them. To say my father showed Art an attitude would be an understatement. He took the opposite side on every issue. There was no logic to his arguments, and no reasoning with him about another point of view. Art quickly learned that the best defense was to keep silent and ignore my father as much as possible. In that silence Art retaliated. When he visited my home, he would read the newspaper or a magazine and essentially ignore my father's attempt at confrontation. It drove my father up the wall.

Discovering the Monster Within

Once, when we were at the bowling alley with my father, Art ordered a beer just for spite. Although he rarely drank anything in those days, Art relished the rare opportunity to make my father squirm. And, Art was a better bowler.

Shortly after our first trip to Johnny Cake, we decided that our parents should meet each other. Mom invited the Burkleys over to the house for a picnic. The idea filled me with dread, but I faced the inevitable with as much verve as I could muster. As usual, my father came through, and my fears were realized.

Art's folks were too kind to tell me what they thought of my parents, but my father quickly informed me that he didn't like Art and Kathleen. They were stuck-up snobs. My mother liked them, but was uncomfortable with their strict set of values, particularly where it concerned the poor. They had little tolerance for the poor, and mom felt we were poor.

In-laws can be a dire influence on young relationships when they don't like each other. But, I believe Art was trying to escape the mold of his family, as much as I was mine. Fortunately, our parent's opinions of each other didn't affect our relationship.

Soon after our parents met each other, I decided to bite the bullet and tell him about my sexual abuse. It took every ounce of courage I could muster. I was certain that when he learned about it, he would run away from me faster than a track star out of the starting blocks. It was that self-worth thing again.

When the time came, I lost most of my nerve. I told him about the abuse and painted it with the broadest possible brush. I couldn't give him explicit details because I couldn't remember any of them. I still can feel the heat of the shame that turned my cheeks scarlet as I bared my soul to him. I was falling in love with Art, and I was so afraid I'd lose him.

After pondering my revelation for a time, Art nodded and assured me that it made no difference at all. He told me that he loved me, and it didn't matter. Besides, he had already met my family, and nothing surprised him.

I shouldn't have been surprised by his response. He had always been so kind and understanding. What I didn't realize was that he lived a very sheltered life, and his knowledge of molestation, sexual abuse and the baggage it carried was more academic than real. He is only now realizing the extent of my ordeal.

For the nursing students, our big party of the year was the prom. The date of the prom my senior year coincided with my twenty-first birthday. I knew it was going to be a special night. Art had already hinted at marriage, and I knew I was in love with him. Still, I wasn't sure I was ready for a life-long commitment. All of ED's arguments raced through my brain. Would I be able to be a good wife? Would I be able to have a normal sexual relationship with him? If we were married, would my life get more out of control? Never once did I doubt I loved him. All the other baggage got in the way.

Before we left for the dance, Art gave me a lovely strand of rose colored cultured pearls. They were the most elegant gift I had ever received. Immediately, my monster told me I didn't deserve them. I knew I didn't, but I was too thrilled not to accept them.

Then, Art asked me to marry him. My heart yearned to say yes, but my brain kept saying no! I trotted out a series of lame excuses. I needed time. I wanted a place of my own. I needed to travel and find out who I was. I told him I loved him but stopped short of saying yes.

Somberly, Art said, "I know. I know exactly how you feel, because I want those same things. Why can't we do them together? We belong together. We both know that."

He was right. My heart told my brain to shut up, and I accepted his proposal. It was the smartest thing I ever did.

The next day, we visited Art's folks. His dad had a number of catalogs strategically placed around the living room open to pages advertising engagement rings. The Burkleys welcomed me into their family with open arms.

My mother was happy for us. My father responded with a grunt. When my sister, Beverly got married, she borrowed a wedding dress, and it broke my mother's heart. She was determined that she would make my wedding dress.

The next weekend, we continued our celebration. Art was living in an apartment in Akron, Ohio, with his roommate, Dan Soloveiko. We arranged a blind date for him with my sister, Linda. It was a beautiful Saturday, and we drove to the Johnny Cake house to pick up Linda. Mom had prepared a beautiful lunch of fried chicken in a wicker picnic basket.

Dan came into the house, and we introduced him to Linda. He sat down on the couch and immediately one of our cats pounced on him.

Wrinkling his nose, Dan blurted out, "I smell cat pee!" We knew at once he would fit right in.

We drove to Euclid Beach Park for the day and had a marvelous time. There was plenty of banter and laughter. Later, we stopped to play miniature golf, and Linda royally skunked Dan, something he was unaccustomed too. I guess he figured any woman who could do that was worth a second look, because they started to date regularly.

I graduated from nurses training that September in the top ten percent of my class. It was one of the proudest days of me life. My parents, and Art's folks were there, and I got to sing in the choir one last time. The sense of accomplishment overwhelmed me, but in the back of my mind, the monster whispered that I was just lucky. As I walked across the stage to get my diploma, I knew in my heart that I had proven my father wrong about what I could do.

Since neither of us had any money, Art and I decided to wait to get married. We eventually planned to get a small apartment, so I went to work saving money. For the time being, I rented a room in the dorm so we could save every cent we could.

Despite the euphoria, I couldn't shake the feeling that I wasn't a hundred percent ready for marriage, so I decided to talk to a counselor at church. Since the first days that mom took us to church, it had been a regular part of my life. I told him about my family, my father's drinking and the abuse. I told him how much I loved, Art, and retold my fears about his size and my commitment. He told me that Art's size was related to my father. I needed someone bigger to protect me from further abuse, and I really didn't need counseling. Then, he told me that I had a very strong survival instinct, so whatever I did I would be fine.

The old boy missed the boat about my father. I wasn't afraid of my father anymore. It was my perception of my own size that was faulty. I felt like a hippo next to a gazelle. That was the problem. He was also wrong about the counseling. I often wonder if he had possessed enough training and experience to diagnose my identity crisis and faulty self-image correctly and had helped me work through that, if I could have been spared decades of torment. He was right about one thing, I am a survivor. I'm a survivor and a fighter, as the next forty years would prove.

Linda and Dan, continued their relationship after the trip to Euclid Beach, and decided that they would get married in the spring, too. A double weeding was out of the question. I wanted my own special day where Art and I would be the center of attention. My mother was beside herself. She couldn't handle two weddings. There wasn't enough money. She couldn't make that many dresses, etc., etc., etc.. Changes would have to be made.

Our wedding date was changed twice. Originally scheduled for spring, this was too close to Linda's and Dan's wedding. First, Art and I thought Christmas time, between the Holidays would be best so Art's sister and her college professor husband could attend. Once again, Mom felt there would be too much to do and too many expenses at Christmas time to do it then. So, we moved it again, this time to November to Mom's satisfaction. Art was all for eloping, but I just couldn't do that to my mother. Why not change? In my own mind, I was still the family outsider. I was the unwanted daughter. Let the daughter they loved and wanted have the choice time. In reality, my mother chose our wedding date for us! One of the most important dates in my life had been dictated by someone else.

My poor fiancé just couldn't understand that kind of compromise. Surprisingly, Art wasn't as angry as he was befuddled. His family wasn't like that, and it took him some time to come to terms with my decision. I couldn't tell him how I felt. Linda was the real daughter, and I was the one they didn't really want. I wasn't worthy enough to fight for my own desires. In the end, as he has always done during our life together, he bit his lip and did what he had to do to make me happy.

There was one humorous fall-out to the change in the date of the wedding. My grandma became convinced that I was pregnant and spread the news around the family like the choice gossip it was. I'm sure she was very disappointed that it wasn't true, though she never mentioned it to me.

Mom and I designed my wedding dress and had a wonderful time shopping for the materials and putting things together. We also made Linda and Beverly's dresses and made and froze an assortment of goodies for the reception. We planned a simple reception with munchies, sandwiches and wedding cake. Despite the logistics, with me in Cleveland, Art working in Akron and Mom in Painesville, we managed to get it all done.

As the pace of preparation accelerated, and the tension developed like steam in a pressure cooker, old ED kept reminding me how fat I would look in my wedding dress if I didn't regularly practice my magic trick. So, I did.

Before the wedding, we went apartment hunting. Art took me to the apartment house where he was living and introduced me to the other guys who lived there. If Art had asked me to make love to him, I'd have gladly accepted his invitation. Ever the gentleman, my kind, safe, rock kept things platonic. I appreciate his behavior a lot more now than I did then.

Once we found a place, we rented a truck and set about moving our furniture. Art's brother, Lew, and my brother, Dave, pitched in to help us. Dave and Lew hit it off and had a wonderful day, working, laughing, cracking jokes and enjoying each other's company. Despite the fun we were having, we had started early in the morning, and it was a long day.

When we were finished, Art drove us all home. We arrived at the Burkley's to drop off Lew well past suppertime. Art's father ordered pizza for us, and I was so hungry I ate some of it over the monster's protest. The tone set earlier in the day by our brothers carried through dinner, and when we left for Johnny Cake to drop off Dave, it was later than we had planned. We piled out of the car in the Archer's driveway like junior high kids flying high. Laughing and giggling we went into the house. Then, the antiaircraft gun opened up and shot us down.

My father exploded in a fit of anger that harkened back to his wet drunk days. He was furious with us. I was so shocked by the hate and rage in his tone that I lapsed into my old disassociative defense. I didn't hear the words he said; I only felt the hatred in them.

It was one of the most humiliating moments of my life. According to my father, we were evil, wicked and had committed an unpardonable sin. We were irresponsible and a host of other invectives. Why? He said it was because we kept Dave out too late. Was that the real reason? Of course it wasn't. Dave was a young adult, and we certainly hadn't damaged him in any way. My father simply seized the opportunity to hurt me. Since I was leaving home for good, he would not have many more opportunities, so he took advantage of every one that came along.

I don't remember the words, but the humiliation is as real to me as it was that night. And, I will never forget Art's magnificent reaction to the horrible attack. Unblinking, he stood there, and faced my father. Already realizing it was useless to argue, Art didn't offer excuses or try to counter the insults. Like a mute, he let my father rave on, and that drove my father to the edge. He wasn't getting to Art, and eventually, my father's wrath was spent in hopeless frustration. With a wave of his hand, he left the field to Art and escaped to his bedroom.

Discovering the Monster Within

As we walked to the car, I held Art's hand in mine. Although his demeanor was calm, there was a barely perceptible tremor in his hand. He didn't say anything at all. Not then, or in the days that followed. The considerable love that I had for him grew more than I thought it could.

We had a small wedding, with about fifty guests. Lew and my sisters and brother were in the wedding. With all the excitement, I had no appetite. ED loved it, but my mother begged me all day to eat, first at breakfast and later at lunch. I ate neither, and ED patted me on the back. I'd look good in that wedding dress.

At promptly four in the afternoon, I walked down the aisle with my father, and he gave me away. Ironically, the man, who caused me the most pain in my life, gave me to the man whose love and devotion in time would help me stop that pain.

After the delightful reception, my mom insisted that we go back to the house and call my grandparents, who couldn't make it to the wedding. Art wasn't sure we should do that, but I coaxed him into it. While we were there, Eva and Donald showed up. By the time we headed for our three-day Niagara Falls honeymoon, it was really late.

We were both exhausted, and the only thing that either of us had eaten was a piece of wedding case. Just across the Pennsylvania line, we scrapped our travel plans and pulled into the Route Nineteen Motel.

Large billboards advertising amateur night should have been posted outside our room. Although Art never wore them, his mother packed him a new pair of pajamas. Kathleen's control over her son reached into our bedroom. It would be the first of many intrusions.

Preparing myself for bed, I used the vaginal cream that was a popular form of contraception then. I was using it because my mother and my mother-in-law said I should. This was my life, but I felt I had no control over it. With a sigh of anticipation and trepidation, I crawled into my marriage bed. Had I not already known that I married a man who would one day be a legitimate candidate for sainthood, the events of the next few hours confirmed it.

The Love of My Life

When we attempted to consummate our marriage, I bled and bled and bled. I was on the verge of tears. I wanted this to be perfect, and my body betrayed me. We were unable to make love. If Art was disappointed, he didn't let it show. He was more concerned with me, and how I felt. I knew I didn't deserve such a man, or such consideration. Once again, I had failed, but, this time, someone was there who cared. Maybe this man was going to make a difference in my life.

The next morning at dawn, Art left our love nest and ventured into a strange town in search of an open store that might sell Kotex. He confided in me later, that while driving the unfamiliar streets that Sunday morning looking for feminine hygiene products, he thought, *"What have I gotten myself into?"* Had he known that ED was along for the honeymoon, he would have had other questions.

When he came back to the motel, he was starved. Except for the bite of cake, neither of us had eaten for twenty-four hours. ED was happy. Art was not. We went to the small café associated with the motel, and Art ordered the entire menu. He had bacon, eggs, toast, cereal, pancakes, home fries, and ate every bite. I joined him and ate a stack of pancakes. ED was furious with me when I didn't bring it back up. I was so delightfully excited I was able to handle the guilt of eating without purging.

For the next three days, as my body healed, we had a grand time at Niagara Falls. And, I continued to dine on such delicacies as hot roast beef sandwiches with mashed potatoes and gravy, and a superb steak dinner. We laughed, talked, and walked hand in hand. I was blissfully happy.

During my healing, Art and I continued to sleep together like brother and sister. He was inordinately patient with me until I was completely healed. As soon as I was, we were able to accomplish what both of us wanted to do that first night, and it was wonderful. And, we have been able to develop a perfectly healthy sex life, despite my abuse. ED, on the other hand, has been a problem.

On the drive home from the Falls, ED whispered in my ear and panic crept over me. Thanksgiving was less than a week away, and I had already eaten enough food to last me for at least six months. I would have to reopen my magic show. ED relaxed and smiled.

I didn't work for the first few days after our wedding, and I had a lot of time to mull over the events of the past week. All doubts about marriage had been erased by Art's love, kindness and gentleness. The way he respected me, and my feelings, was beyond my comprehension. I knew that I was the luckiest woman alive, and that I didn't deserve it. Just like I didn't deserve to be in the Archer family, I didn't deserve to be this wonderful man's wife. But, I would work hard to be the best wife I could, and maybe one day, I could make myself worthy.

The stage was set for my monster to grow. My life's ambition was accomplished, and I had the nursing degree to prove it. The urge to wave it in my father's face and say, "I told you so," was strong. But, I resisted. I had just gotten married to a wonderful man, who was loving and protective and respected me for who I was. I should have been the happiest woman in the world. Still, I felt woefully inadequate.

For most of my life, I have been a mirror, reflecting what others saw there, and not feeling in control of anything in my life. Even though Art accepted me as I was, I couldn't see that. Each word of encouragement, each attempt at building my sense of worth was distorted by the way I interpreted his comments and those of others around me. When inadequacy dominates your life, you always feel out of control. Eating disorders are about control. Nearly everyone I have met with an eating disorder shared that diminished sense of who they are and what they were worth. What we eat is the one thing that we feel we can completely control, so we do.

A peculiar facet of the ED personality is its complete lack of culinary boundaries. I never knew if I was full or hungry. If I were hungry, I might have to eat. If I had to eat, I might lose control, so it was safer not to eat. I thought I was in complete control of what I ate, but I wasn't. I never realized that I had crossed the line, and my monster was now in control. I was still out of control but with a monster at the helm. ED skillfully hid that little detail from me.

The Love of My Life

One of my first failures in marriage concerned food. I couldn't cook, and I didn't know it. Mom had always done the family's cooking, so I never paid much attention to that. Oh, I helped here and there, but since I had little interest in the table, I never got actively involved in the preparation.

My first attempt at a big meal involved roasted chicken that ended up bloody in the center and burned on the outside. When I tried a pot roast, it was so tough our jaws locked with fatigue trying to chew it. Determined not to fail my husband, I attacked cookbooks the same way I had my nursing texts. Despite not enjoying the food myself, I became a pretty fair cook. When we entertained, my guests often had seconds and always complimented me on the results of my labor.

Instead of taking the compliments the way I should have, praise made me feel guilty. I really wasn't a cook. I was only following cookbook directions. Anybody could do that. I forced myself to cook out of self defense. I didn't deserve any accolades. ED loved that attitude, and reminded me what I was really good at.

Since I felt I had no worth, I displayed another of the classic characteristics of the inadequate personality. I allowed Art to become the complete focus of my life. My emotions became mirror images of his. If he was happy, I was happy. If he was sad, I was sad. He paid the bills, handled the money, made the major decisions and planned our leisure activities. After all, I had no opinion, and even if I did, mine were valueless. By trying, in my distorted way, to be a devoted wife, I was digging the hole of disrespect for myself deeper.

In the first decade of our marriage, I never disagreed with Art. If I felt his decision or opinion was less than perfect, I swallowed my bile, even if it choked me. Unfortunately, I allowed it to fester inside. Years of these self-imposed toxins later erupted and nearly poisoned our relationship.

ED was ecstatic. This was exactly what he wanted. Since I had given up everything else in my life, control of food was all that was left, and he assured me that I was doing a great job with that.

Discovering the Monster Within

We moved into our apartment in Cuyahoga Falls, a suburb of Akron, and began the typical life of so many young married couples. Working hard, we saved every penny for a down payment on our dream house.

I worked four days a week on a medical floor. Since we only had one car, on my work days, I dropped Art at the bus stop and kept the car. Of course, this bothered me. I fretted about him being out in the cold, the rain, the snow, or having to wait too long for the bus. I should have been doing that, not Art. So, I tried to make up for it.

Keeping the tiny apartment tidy was no problem. I worked on my cooking and quickly found Art's favorites then cooked them as often as I dared. I turned to baking, and mastered Art's sister's pie crust and Mom's sweet rolls. Of course I didn't eat any of it. In fact, I cooked without ever tasting anything.

I was always careful about my appearance, but since I was so fat, I had to lose a few more pounds. I weighed a whopping one hundred thirteen pounds on my wedding day, and that was way too much. I needed to be slim and trim to please my man.

While we lived in the apartment, we went house hunting with Linda and Dan.. It was a bitter day, and the cold turned the roads to streams of frigid slush. Puddles of icy water dotted the bleak landscape like moon craters. The cold of the Ohio winter seeped into my marrow like battery acid into metal. Despite that, I refused to dress sensibly or wear boots. Being so fat and unattractive, I had to do everything I could to look good.

Returning to the car after a viewing, Art looked at me with some annoyance.

"Pat, your face is dirty," he growled. "Don't you know enough to wash your face before you go out?"

I was crushed. Fighting back tears, I gazed into the rearview mirror at my dusky face. Retrieving a handkerchief from my purse, I wiped at the offending color. It didn't come off. My face wasn't dirty; it was dusky with cyanosis from the cold. That eased my humiliation. To be freezing, rather than dirty, was the better option.

The Love of My Life

When they realized the true reason for my dirty face, they began to fuss over me and took me straight home to warm up. The guilt settled in on the ride to the apartment. I ruined the house hunt, and allowed myself to be at the mercy of the weather. They were all upset with me; they were just being too polite to show it. Once more things were out of control. Out of control! "No, no cocoa; just black coffee please."

As I got to know Art's family better, they became another problem for me. They impressed upon me their educational standards which included no sympathy for slackers. Personal appearance was high on their list, and when I was around them, I was overly conscious about how I looked. Furthermore, fat was not on their radar screen. Fat was a mortal sin. Fat was from the Devil. Since I was fat, that was a constant source of anxiety for me.

Also on their agenda was financial security, and Art had been inoculated with a full dose of that vaccine. The financial position of the family, no matter how secure, was of major concern to them. If they had ten dollars, they needed twenty. If they had possessed a million, they would have needed two. I was firmly convinced that I could never truly be a part of their family. I could never meet their expectations.

I was terrified that my relationship with the Burkleys would cause my marriage to fail. So I doubled my efforts to please everyone else. Once again, I was the outsider trying to prove to my family that I belonged, just as I had done as a child.

On the brighter side, as we approached our first anniversary, we found the little house at four hundred Madison Avenue. And, to our joy, I was pregnant.

Unfortunately, I miscarried very early. My dream was dashed. I had failed at one of the most important things in my married life. ED had already started to take his toll on my health, and my gynecologist told me that I wasn't strong enough to work and carry children, too. Shortly thereafter, Art and I decided I should stop work, and we would try to have a child.

Discovering the Monster Within

After I stopped working, my old friend guilt called. I could hear my father's voice in the back of my mind, though I did my best to keep it from my conscious thought. I was living up to his negativity, quitting work after such a short time to have babies. I could see the, "I told you so," look in his eyes. Fortunately, since Art and my father had such enmity for each other, I seldom saw him. Besides, I had already convinced myself this was only temporary. I'd go back to work one day soon.

Worse than that, since I'd already lost one pregnancy, I didn't know if I could carry a child, even if I was able to get pregnant again. Art had given me so much happiness and security that I was determined to give him a child.

CHAPTER 7

Kids and ED

Little is written concerning anorexia and pregnancies. The reason is simple. Most anorexics do not have menstrual periods, signaling a lack of ovulation. We effectively sterilize ourselves. Another reason is that we are so consumed by eating behaviors that the thoughts of having a child are beyond the scope of our radar.

As has been the course of my life, I was different in this regard. Despite now being in the throws of significant anorexia, I was hell bent to have children. Having a degree in nursing helped me. I knew just enough about the nutrition of pregnancy to be dangerous. But, I could control my eating, so I reasoned that I could eat healthy enough to carry a child if I wanted too.

This pattern of intellectual disassociation is so close to the emotional type I practiced during my father's attacks that transference was simple. I could envision things as though I was on the outside looking in at a white rat in an experimental box. It was as if what I was doing made logical, intellectual sense, and the consequences of my behavior were unintelligible to me. With that faulty tape playing in my head, I set about to have a family.

Discovering the Monster Within

Since I had stopped working, with my energy levels and so much time on my hands I had been able to perfect my eating habits. Mom never ate breakfast, so neither did I. In time, I could talk myself out of being hungry. There was always something else to do to keep from eating. I'll eat after I vacuum; after I do the ironing; after I weed the garden. Within a few weeks, I felt less hungry. I was in complete control of my intake, and ED patted me on the back.

Another ploy honed to perfection was my Jack-in-the-box technique. I always cooked for others, and truly enjoyed entertaining. If I talked a lot, fussed with the presentation of the food and popped up and down, like a Jack-in-the box, to fill a water glass, get more potatoes, or check on something on the stove, I never had to eat.

My one sin during this period was ice cream. I used my bulimic binge and purge behavior to expunge myself, and always with an eye on the scale.

The day my period was late, I had to fight to contain myself. I wanted to hope but was afraid to. When the doctor told me I was pregnant, I literally floated home. Somehow, I had convinced myself that the only reason Art married me was so he could have children. Now, I had a chance to make him really happy. This time, I wouldn't fail.

When I told him, he was as happy as I was. Yet, in the edges of his eyes, I could see he shared my fears. I interpreted his mood to say he was afraid I might fail, too. My faulty interpretive skills were now well developed. For one glorious evening, we put those fears aside to bask in the joy of the moment.

Later that night, as Art snored contentedly on the pillow beside me, sleep was elusive. I couldn't slow the parade of anxiety that marched across my mind like a circus animals. Art was still too small, and I felt too fat. My role in the extended family remained cloudy. What would happen if I was not able to carry this child either? Would they expel me from the family? Would I ever really be a part of Art's life if I couldn't give him children?

Kids and ED

Over the next few days, a grim reality settled over me. The pregnancy was going to be a monumental challenge for me. My desire to have this child overwhelmed any concern about my size, my appearance or my own health. I pushed ED into a closet in my mind and slammed the door. Yet, every time I let down my guard for a second, he nudged the door open and nagged and nagged and nagged.

My first task was to inventory the foods necessary to have a healthy baby and lay in a goodly supply of them. I discerned what foods were healthy and would put little to no weight on my frame. They became my staples. Because they were needed by the child, I forced myself to eat things I usually wouldn't. As the guilt and anxiety over eating threatened to drive me to the toilet bowl, I would close my eyes and image a newborn baby in my arms. Using this imagery, I was able to control the adverse impulses.

I handled stress, change and emotions the same way I did as a child. I was never emotional, and seldom ever cried. A crying female was proof positive that my father's view of women was correct. With each crisis, I buried my emotions, subjugated my feelings and gradually allowed ED to convince me that it was noble to take the blame for everything that went wrong. My wants and wishes were unimportant, he told me. It's for the good of the order.

In the fourth month of the pregnancy, the spotting and bleeding began. I was so frightened that I was afraid my heart would stop beating. As the doctors ordered me to bed, the victim in me responded true to form. What had I done? Had I eaten the right things? Had I restricted too much? Whatever the problem was, I caused it. Biting my lip to hold back the tears I refused to shed, I agonized over the likelihood of another failure. What would I do if I failed again? The darkness I had fantasized about as a child returned.

Fortunately, the bleeding stopped, and five months later, when the first pangs of labor struck me, I was ecstatic. I arrived at Saint Thomas Hospital in Akron for what proved to be a prolonged stay. Labor then lacked a number of today's civilities. I was in a room alone. It had no windows and no nurse's call light, but the nurses looked in frequently. Although Art was right down the hall in the waiting room (husbands, parents, video cameras and heaven knows what else were not allowed in the delivery room at the time), I have never felt so alone.

As labor snailed along, the doctors told me it would be at least two or three in the morning before our child would be born. And, we had a dog. The doctor told Art to go home and take care of the poor animal. By then, my parents had arrived, so it would be alright. Art's aunt, his mother's sister had passed away, and his folks were attending the funeral out of state. They missed all the excitement.

Despite the fact that the doctor had told Art it would be fine to go, and it was the right thing to do for the poor dog, my parents were furious when he left. Poor Art was half way home when my membranes ruptured. At ten forty-five in the evening, hours before the doctor's prediction, on May fourteenth, nineteen sixty-five, our daughter, Carolyn, was born.

Art didn't make it back until shortly after she was born. He had just returned to the hospital as I exited the elevator on my way from the delivery room to my hospital room. I told him we had a baby girl, and he kissed me before they wheeled me to my room. My parents were livid that Art had "missed" the event. It really didn't matter, because they never let any of them see me or the baby for a full hour after that. But my parents never forgave him. They found an imaginary spot on Prince Charming's coat and they were not about to let him forget it.

When we brought our daughter home from the hospital, it was my turn to be livid. Art was playing on a softball team, and they had a game that evening. He took Carolyn and me home, settled us in and headed for the game. My warped interpretation of events made me ask myself what I had done wrong. Why does he *have* to play ball tonight? Doesn't he love me? Doesn't he love the baby? What did I say? What did I do to drive him away? A new baby is an adjustment for any couple; I needed Art with me tonight.

Kids and ED

Then, my old buddy ED popped up to remind me that I was nothing but a baby factory anyhow. I didn't deserve special consideration. Just shut up and do my job. So, I did.

Art came home from the game on crutches. He had torn a ligament in his left knee. Some wives, and in some way a more normal response, might have been to give a rousing cheer at his predicament. It served him right for running out on me and our new baby. Of course, I couldn't begin to think of it that way. Had my desire to have him home with me caused the injury? Had something I did or said make him lose concentration and get hurt? It was my fault; my fault. When I write it now, it sounds so stupid, but that night, it's exactly what I was thinking.

With the injury, Art had a terrible time with stairs, and I wasn't allowed to do them yet. The diaper pail was upstairs and the washer and dryer in the basement. Risking life and limb, Art teetered down the stairs and waited while I rinsed the dirty diapers and tossed them down to him. He waited there to wash and dry the soiled linens and toss the clean ones back to me before hobbling back up the stairs again. Disposable diapers, which had not yet been introduced, would have deprived us of all that fun.

My most cherished moments of those first few months were those Art and I spent at the side of her crib watching her sleep. This tiny miracle was the product of our love, and it thrilled us beyond measure. Standing there, with Art's hand in mine, I made a solemn vow to shower this child with the love, warmth and affection I had never felt as a child. Her life would be different. I would see to that!

As soon as I recovered from the effects of the delivery, I returned to my old eating habits. Purging became a frequent event, yet I felt hungrier than I ever had. I found myself eating in the middle of the night. I discovered that if I froze a fig bar, it took longer to eat it. The combination of the corrosive effects of the stomach acid and frozen fig bars took their toll on my genetically inferior teeth ushering in decades of dental work. And, no dentist ever questioned my eating habits.

Discovering the Monster Within

There is a sign most physicians and dentists I have talked to are unaware of that is a tip off for bulimic behavior. It's called Russel's sign. When self-induced vomiting is promulgated by sticking one's fingers down one's throat, the constant abrasion of the teeth against the knuckles or the back of the hand causes ridges or calluses to form. Since my bulimic behavior was never initiated in that fashion, I didn't develop the sign, but I had enough other symptoms that should have been picked up. Perhaps they were but the doctors and dentists didn't know what to do about my disease.

We had lived in a comfortable little house on Madison Avenue for several years when our next door neighbor got his real estate license. On a whim, we put our house up for sale, and to our surprise and dismay the house sold immediately. My stress levels skyrocketed. What were we going to do? Where were we going to live? We didn't have any friends to watch the now six month old Carolyn while we got ready to move. ED stepped forward and helped me eat almost nothing while we house hunted.

We found a big old house on Ohio Street to rent until we found something to buy. In November, we moved in. At that time, we were attending The First United Methodist Church in Cuyahoga Falls. To our delight, Ed Thorn, the assistant minister, and his wife Eldora with their boys, five year old Carson and four year old Michael, lived next door. They became the first really good friends of our married life and remain so to this day.

Once we settled in, I relegated ED to the basement of my life temporarily. I couldn't resist the occasional purge, but that was under extreme circumstances. I had learned to restrict my intake to control my weight, and that's all I had to do. When Eldora and I stopped for lunch on our frequent shopping excursions, I began to eat salads (no dressing) for lunch, a habit that lasted the next thirty-five years. I could push the lettuce around, play with the tomato and nibble on the celery with its negative calories. All the while I kept up a stream of chatter so she wouldn't notice how much I wasn't eating.

Kids and ED

Those eight months we spent on Ohio Street were simply delightful. Since my literary education had been sorely neglected, I read Crime and Punishment and other classics and became an Agatha Christie fan. I worked at sewing and baking and enjoying Carolyn. We celebrated her first birthday with the Thorns, a party I still recall with fondness.

Although I enjoyed the respite, ED kept nudging my guilt levels about not working. I was doing what my father said I would. I had my baby and I wasn't working.

The following spring, we found the house that would be our home until we retired. A tidy little cape on Bancroft Street in Cuyahoga Falls, it was situated on a dead end street with a lot that backed up to a city park. It was perfect.

Immediately, my yin and yang started in on me. I was secure, happy and safe on Ohio Street with dear friends next door. Why should we move? Did I really want to move? Art did, and since I marched to his drum, I accepted the upcoming move and swallowed my feelings. The apprehension ratcheted up my anxiety levels to the breaking point,, until ED stepped in and helped me ease the tension by eating less and regaining control of my out of control emotions.

On July fourth, we moved into our new home, and five months later I was pregnant again. I immediately reinstituted the routine that had worked with Carolyn, eating the things that would be good for the baby and not fattening for me. I was now down to a svelte one hundred three pounds breeder who was proving she could do it all.

I didn't want to binge when we went out to eat. That would be unacceptable. So, I began to eat healthy things at home before leaving and practically nothing when we were out. ED issued me a passing mark.

My second pregnancy was uneventful until the very end. My life was structured, and I felt content. I was giving Art another child which validated my worth to him. I had become the model domestic, complete with gardening and fine cuisine. Just like my father told me I would. Damn!

Discovering the Monster Within

We got together frequently with new friends Tom and Linda Reed during this time, and I was introduced to a wonderful new game called bridge. Art never played games like Risk or Monopoly, but card games, especially bridge, fascinated him. With his mathematical mind, he is an awesome bridge player. Much to my surprise, I liked it too. I spent hours reading Goren on Bridge and playing and studying the hands in the book. I was hooked. It gave me a great feeling of accomplishment, and I became very good at it. I frequently deferred to my partners, even if they were inferior players. Still, I played every chance I got. We had some bridge nuts at church and our neighbors Chuck and Alice Ferrell played. I still enjoy the game, but even more now. I can be myself, and take control when the situation dictates that I do so. That feels good.

My due date for the second pregnancy was August twenty-ninth, but of course, I couldn't do things the easy way. The first of August, both Carolyn and Art were sick with fevers and gastrointestinal distress. That night, I went into labor.

With no one else to call, I called the old ob-clinic nurse, Art's mom. It was five in the morning, but I had no other choice. I told her I had been in labor since three. As we talked, Art's dad woke up and began chastising her.

"You talk on the phone all day long, and now you're up in the middle of the night doing it. Give it a rest!" he grumbled.

Telling him about my labor, she dressed and roared from Cleveland to Cuyahoga Falls, about a forty minute trip. She decided immediately that I needed to go to the hospital. Bundling me into the car, she drove me to the emergency room door, dropped me off and sped back to the house to take care of the rest of my family, who were too sick to get out of bed.

I stepped from the sidewalk into an emergency room nightmare. It started with the admitting nurse.

"Where's your husband? Isn't anybody with you?" she said acidly.

"No, I'm by myself, and my contractions are very close together," I replied, gritting my teeth and trying to remain civil.

"You don't look pregnant," another nurse chimed in.

"I am, and I'm terribly uncomfortable," I said, beginning to lose my composure.

"You don't look uncomfortable. Here, fill these out," she said, shoving insurance papers at me.

Instead of telling her to take the papers and shove them, I painfully filled them out. They finally took me into the exam room. When they found how far along I was, the chaos began. Mostly, they shouted at me for waiting so long to come in. At least that was my perception of the conversation, and this time, I believe it is was an accurate translation of the facts.

In a sequence straight from the Keystone Cops, we raced down the hall. They flopped me onto the delivery table and barely got the spinal in. Fortunately, natural childbirth wasn't in vogue then. All four pounds twelve ounces of David Lewis Burkley slipped into the world on August second, nineteen sixty-seven. The birth weight was lower than Carolyn's. Apparently I didn't do as good a job with nutrition on this pregnancy.

Following the delivery, I bled. I bled a great deal, and they kept me in the delivery room for a long time. When they wheeled me out, Mom and my brother Dave had arrived. I can't tell you how happy I was to see them.

Three weeks early, David continued to lose weight until he was down to four pounds seven ounces. My anxiety titer went up. Was it my fault? They kept him in the hospital for another week until he reached five pounds. Every day, Art, drove me back to the hospital so I could hold him and feed him. I didn't nurse any of the children because I was sustaining my body only enough to keep them healthy during pregnancy. Nursing them was never part of the equation. I realized these things, but I gave no thought to what I was doing to my own body with such irrational behavior.

I had my other problems post-partum. Severe attacks of what they diagnosed as gallbladder pain wracked my body during pregnancy. When they worked up the problem after delivery, they found a gastric ulcer. Standard ulcer therapy in nineteen sixty-seven consisted of Maalox and half-and-half. It was ghastly, especially for someone who hadn't eaten anything as rich as half-and-half in years. I could hardly get the loathsome liquid down. To compensate, I adjusted my diet. Fortunately, I was too apprehensive about the ulcer to do much purging.

My father came to see David the third day after he was born. Dad was having problems breathing and had been diagnosed with emphysema. There was a haunted look in his eyes, and he did something totally unexpected. He confessed he was afraid, because they told him they had to do other tests. He was living the prophecy he had made so many times when I was a child.

"It makes no difference. I won't live much past fifty anyhow," he had told us.

When the test results were in, he was diagnosed with far advanced multiple myeloma, an aggressive cancer of the blood and lymphatic system. The prognosis was three to six months.

My mother called me with the news. She decided not to tell my father his prognosis. It was totally her decision. I'm not sure if it was the right one or not. We spent the rest of his life pretending he was going to recover, and he spent the rest of his life looking into our eyes and knowing we were lying to him.

As a nurse, I saw many people whose families tried that ploy, and believe me, they were fooling nobody. More that one patient has said to me, "My wife (or husband or child) keeps telling me I'm going to get better, but I know I'm not. If it makes them feel better to act that way, I won't spoil their little game."

It was not long before my father realized the inevitable. His death was horrendous, and he was at home for most of it, bed ridden and terrified. He wouldn't give my mother a moment's peace. Requiring constant attention, he would call out to her like a child in fear of the closet monster if she was out of the room for five minutes.

Kids and ED

Once, in sheer desperation, she called me in the middle of the night and held the phone down by his bed so I could hear his agonizing screams. The pure wretchedness of it made my blood run cold. The cancer had eaten into his bones, and the slightest movement caused him distilled misery and wracked his frail body with pain. What should she do? Since 911 was still a decade away, I told her to call an ambulance and get him some help.

His remaining time was spent in and out of the hospital. Each time, he grew weaker. One of the last times we saw him, he was propped up in one of those old-fashioned wooden wheelchairs, looking like a living cadaver. He wanted to hold his new grandson one last time. I laid David in his arms, and for a moment, I could smell the fragrance of a plastic corsage.

Because his illness was so terrible, when the end came, we greeted it with relief. I don't harbor any repressed grief over his passing. When he died, I felt no anger, no guilt. I pitied the terrible pain of his last days, but there was no malicious revenge in that pity. No matter what he had done, no one, not even an animal, deserves to die the way he did.

Did I love him? Did I grieve? The answer to both questions is yes. He was, after all, my father, and not everything he did for his children was terrible. His appalling actions dominate the memories, making it difficult to remember the rest of the man. I felt sorry for him; that his life had been so hard, and that he never had an opportunity to live and love in a nurturing environment. I also felt sorry for myself, because I never had the type of relationship that a daughter should have with her father. All those who mourn wish the dead to rest in peace. I hope my father rests in peace, because his entire life was spent at war with himself, his fellow man and, in particular, with those cared about him.

When I was finally able to bring David home, it was an enormous sense of accomplishment. I *was* a good wife. I hadn't let Art down. I had given him a daughter and a son. I was a success.

Unfortunately, Carolyn wasn't ready for competition. I tried to compensate for it by doing special things both with and for her. I made her clothes, bought her little presents, spent extra time doting on her, and I made certain she had a grand birthday party every year. I was determined to give her the love and security I never had in life. Although I know I did that, I'm not sure I succeeded in making her life any happier.

David was hyperactive and cursed with a series of gruesome ear infections that left us in fear for his hearing. Despite all our attempts, Carolyn continued to develop a dominating personality. Once, for example, Carolyn hid David in the closet while he was in his walker. After searching frantically for him, I found him playing among the coats as if nothing had happened. David took it most of the time, but when his patience was exhausted, he fought back with the fury that is unique to hyperactive children.

I tried to be earth mother, fight referee, loving companion and pediatric nurse, but sometimes I was overwhelmed. In an attempt to regain some semblance of control in my life, I concentrated on the area ED and I knew I could control. I continued to ignore breakfast and started skipping lunches as well. There was plenty to do, so I could stay busy enough to avoid eating. If I felt hungry, I talked myself out of it. Retrospectively, I wonder where I found the energy to keep going.

Nearing David's first birthday, I was pregnant again, triggering another crisis with Art's folks. They were extremely critical of my condition and informed me that this was too soon for me to be pregnant again. My health would be ruined. The baby might end up with problems. They never said those things directly, but the less-than subtle message was there. Were the comments prompted by my eating habits? I don't know, but shortly following their dire predictions, I miscarried.

The next time Art's folks visited us, they informed me that it was for the best. I never totally forgive them for that comment, but it reinforced an indelible lesson. Take off the rose colored glasses when you deal with others, be they friend, foe or relative.

Despite her early pushes to get us together, Art's mom never really added the personal touches that would have made me feel at ease. For example, I never received a birthday or Christmas present from her.

It was always an impersonal check made out to Mr. and Mrs. Arthur Burkley.

With each check, the monster stirred the pot. ED told me the reason she did it was because I was worth nothing to her. Writing out a check fulfilled her social obligation and kept us in balance with the gifts to her other children. The monster suggested to me that if I weren't so fat, she might like me better. After all, the Burkley's didn't like fat women.

On the other hand, Art's dad always got me a little personal something every Christmas. It made me feel special. One of his last presents was a blue cloth bathrobe that I wore until the material in the sleeves disintegrated.

Christmas caused my two-edged sword to whistle through the air. Decorating the house, baking Christmas cookies I wasn't going to eat, and buying gifts was a joy. But, the silent conflicts between our two families cast a pall over the celebration.

I felt guilty when Art's parents spent more on us than my folks did. My parents didn't help the situation. They never missed an opportunity to tell me that they could never measure up to the Burkley's

Art developed a maddening habit of keeping a separate list for each child, with an accurate accounting of the number of presents and amounts spent for each child. They had to be identical. This never computed with me, and I just couldn't understand it. The conflict in my mind about the monetary value placed on Christmas grew with the years.

The pattern continued, and he showered the children with clothes, shoes, the best musical instruments and college tuition. Having worked for everything I ever got in my life, I felt sad that the children never had an opportunity to feel the sense of accomplishment that came from earning some of it themselves. When I asked Art about it, he replied, "Why is your way of showing love right, and my way of showing it wrong?"

I was not equipped to accept his statement as anything but a criticism of me, so I did. How I wish I had realized, that Art, like me, was a product of his environment, and that I should understand it and not allow it to warp what I did with my life. How much easier it would have made things. Those were the values that had been instilled in him. That's how his parents handled things, and he was simply following his genes.

The same is true of his attitude around the holidays. My loving, gentle husband becomes irritable, sad, depressed and walks about smoldering with barely repressed anger. All my life I accepted that as my fault. I wasn't pleasing him; wasn't a good enough wife; wasn't a good enough mother. It took me over forty years to lovingly approach him about it.

When I did, he was really good about it. He explained that he feels responsible for the holidays. He has to be certain everyone else has a great time. The internal pressure he places upon himself is enormous. It overwhelms him, and he gets angry with himself because he feels he's not doing a good enough job.

All those years I thought it was me, me, me. It wasn't me. Art was human and had concerns of his own. I never bothered to look for them or try to help him address them. Thank God I have some of the skills to handle these things, now; I only wish I had them forty years sooner.

When I became pregnant again, I guess Art's folks felt I was beyond hope, because they didn't make much of it this time. I thought if I could give Art four children, then I would be as good as my mother.

In the late sixties, most obstetricians harped on weight gain during pregnancy, the limit being twenty pounds. Although I took care of myself in the early going, I chewed a lot of gum and kept frantically busy. I restricted foods that would not be good for the baby.

At six and a half months, we invited our friends, Tom and Linda Reed, over to play bridge. It's strange how the brain freezes sentinel events like photographs that can be viewed from the mind's album on demand. I had just finessed the queen of diamonds to make the contract and win the rubber. Laughing and joking, I was flushed with success when I suddenly wet my pants. Or so I thought, until I saw the crimson stain soaking through my dress.

Kids and ED

Our friends stayed with the children while Art rushed me to the hospital. The doctors worked like demons, but had a hard time controlling the hemorrhage and premature labor. They transfused me, started an intravenous alcohol drip and sedated me with Seconal, to no avail. Our second son, Dennis, was born on November first, nineteen sixty-nine. So premature that his lungs had not fully developed, our son was transferred to Akron Children's Hospital.

My aching mouth, full of sutures from recent dental surgery added to my discomfort. After a long, dreadful night, the day dawned gray and mournful, as if nature was already lamenting my impending loss. My pediatrician came into the room with the expression of an undertaker on his face.

"Pat, there's no gentle way to say this. Your baby is going to die. I'm sorry," he said. Later, Art, who had been called at home about 6:00 a.m. and informed of the baby's death, came into the room dressed in a suit. He didn't have to say anything. I knew that our son was gone.

Mom and Ray, mom's new husband, and Tom and Linda Reed, who had also lost a child, were lifesavers in my sea of grief. I never saw my little boy. I never touched him, held him, or told him I loved him. Although I felt as if my heart would crush under the weight of sadness, I didn't grieve. I handled this crisis as I did all the others in my life. I disassociated myself from the feelings, internalized them and went on with my life.

Over the years, I went to the gravesite only once. Though he frequently came to my mind, Dennis was a phantom child to me. Since I'd never seen him, I couldn't even put a face with his memory. Art, who *had* seen him, never visited the grave at all. He handled the loss in his way. The child was gone, and if he behaved as though Dennis had never lived at all, he could cope with his heartbreaking loss.

When we retired, and were leaving Ohio, I asked Art to take me to the cemetery. As we stood there in the sunlight, the bottled up grief rolled down my cheeks as rivers of tears. Holding my hand, Art wept with me. Only then were we at peace with the memory of the son who might have been.

We decided to pursue birth control, so I talked to Art's sister about diaphragms.

She had tried them but was less than thrilled. Her advice was to put it in at night and take it out in the morning. Even though I didn't like the idea, I decided to try one.

I used it faithfully, putting it in at night and taking it out in the morning. My next pregnancy was conceived in mid-morning, when I didn't have the diaphragm in. Why didn't I stop and put it in? Did I subconsciously forget it on purpose? Did the passion of the moment overcome common sense? I really don't know. I do know that when I found I was pregnant again, I felt elated, petrified and guilty, all at the same time.

Since my gynecologist had told me not to get pregnant again, I was in a quandary. In those days, the only place abortions were done was New York. I really didn't want an abortion. Art was the only one I could talk to about it but he was as torn as I was. In the end, he told me that I was the one risking my health, and the decision would have to be mine.

Still in the first trimester, Art and I went out to dinner. Despite guilt that I had in some way harmed Dennis with my eating, I was back on my standard feed-the-baby starve-the-mother diet. At the end of my meager emotional resources, I told Art that regardless of the cost, I was going to have this baby. I gave him the options of taking the children and leaving, or I would move out. He didn't have to go through the ordeal. If he wanted, I'd give him an uncontested divorce; whatever it took to ease his mind. It was obvious from my illogical choices that my emotional well was dry.

Looking across the table, a broad grin creased his boyish face. "No, *we* will have this child," he said.

Is it any wonder that I love the man?

Kids and ED

My due date was March fifteenth, income tax day in the seventies. To give myself the best chance to carry the child, I worked my diet to perfection, eased the restrictive behavior and resisted all ED's urging to purge. As has been the pattern of my life, when I see a light at the end of the tunnel it turns out to be a train.

My brother, Dave, had met his future wife Suzanne, and they were living in different states. While undertaking a long term romance, they contemplated marriage. Somehow, they arrived at the brilliant conclusion that if they moved to Ohio, one of them could live with us and the other with Dan and Linda. That way, they could date more regularly and decide about their future together. Linda heard about it first and snatched Dave. Passing the buck to us, we were placed in the awkward position of either accepting or rejecting Suzanne.

Art was livid. We had two little ones, and the pregnancy with its associated dangers. He felt his space was being forcefully invaded, and he wanted no part of it. I was torn, because if I said no to the family, it would be a huge problem. They reassured me it would only be for a short time. Seeing my pain and turmoil, Art agreed she could stay with us.

It was not a good time for a houseguest, and she wasn't particularly helpful to me. One night, she cooked liver and onions for my brother. We thought it was health food back then. The dirty dishes were left in the sink soaking in water overnight, dripping with grease. When I discovered them the next morning, the sight nauseated me. It was all I could do to reach into the sink and pull them out. I had no problem restricting that morning.

The stress of her being there was nearly intolerable, and the victim in me relished it. Keeping strictly to my diet, I had additional things to do to keep me busy. Jack-in-the-box was there for every meal, and I had no problem staying under the twenty pound minimum obstetricians harped on.

In retrospect, Suzanne was only with us for a short time. She gave me an excuse to occasionally let ED out of solitary confinement and gave me something else to fret about, taking my mind off the dangers of my pregnancy. The secondary gain of service to the family stroked both my ego and the victim in me.

On New Year's Eve only six months into my pregnancy, I went into labor for the first time. Demons leaped from my subconscious to ask me if it was going to start all over again. That was one time I was glad I had never seen Dennis. If I had, he would have marched from the grave to rattle chains at me. Still, the specter of another dead child hung over me like a summer thundercloud. Oddly, I had no concern for my own safety. This time, the doctors stopped the labor.

The episodic labor became a pattern. Each time I was ready to leave the hospital, it would snow heavily between the time Art left to pick me up and the time we returned home. He would drop me off at our neighbors, shovel the snow off the hill on our driveway so the car could make it up, pick me up and drive me home. It got to be a joke. Our neighbor, Martha LaGuardia, was a Godsend for me. No matter the time of day or night, she took Carolyn and David under her wing and mothered them until I came back.

At the hospital, they always sedated me and started the alcohol drip, standard therapy for premature labor in a world where fetal alcohol syndrome was twenty years away. Art thought my slurred speech was hilarious and offered to bring me olives or a twist. The doctors planned to take the fetus to a viable weight and then do a Cesarean Section.

On February twenty-fifth, nineteen seventy one, Art and I became the proud parents of a five pound one-half ounce bouncing baby boy. Art and my mom were there for the section. Now, it was time to name our boy. Children's names had not come easy for us. Carolyn waited three days for a first name and never did get a middle name, because we couldn't agree.

Names are very important for Art. He was dead set against any juniors. I loved the name Diane for a girl, but that was over the line for Art. That bothered me. Diana was a beautiful Greek goddess. Why couldn't our daughter have that name? We compromised on Carolyn.

I had been fond of the name David, not so much because of my brother, but because of David in the Bible. He was a strong, principled, dashing hero, whose name slipped poetically from the tongue. Our son could do worse than have his namesake. It was Art's first choice. And, he wanted the middle name to be Lewis. He would be named after both brothers.

With this pregnancy, the name game started again in earnest. We had so much trouble with the name that we came to the irrational conclusion that if it was a boy, he would name it, and I would have nothing to say about the name. If it was a girl, I would name it and he would have no input. I had named Dennis, since Art couldn't bring himself to name a dead child. It was another way Art dealt with Dennis' death.

It was one of the dumbest pacts of our married life. As Art became more fixated with finding a name, I became less convinced that it mattered. The child who would grow and develop was the important thing, not the name, as long as it wasn't an embarrassing tag that would shame the child the rest of his days.

When Art marched into the room and told me the child's name would be Calvin Arthur after his two grandfathers, I was dumbfounded! He explained that there would be confusion if he reversed the names, and the kid would be saddled with a nick name. As the decision sunk in, an eerie feeling pervaded me as I contemplated the distaste Art had for my father.

Unfortunately, at this point in our relationship, if Art and I didn't discuss a potential problem, it didn't exist. I didn't bring up my concerns about the name and its implications. He didn't say anything else about it either.

The good wife syndrome played a part in this decision. I buried my wishes, desires and opinions in deference to Art's. His word was law, and I never challenged it. Besides, I was stuck with this stupid deal. We had a son, and it was Art's right to name him.

I prayed about it, and talked to myself about not attaching my father's personality or actions to my son's name. I would honor my husband and love my son. It was the right thing to do, and time has vindicated my decision.

The competent psychologist would say that naming the boys David and Calvin gave me a chance to remake my dysfunctional family into a new, unflawed one. Thank God that's not true. Regardless, my two young men have given those names their own wonderful interpretation. I love both of them and their names.

Following Calvin's birth, I had a tremendous problem with water retention and my periods abruptly ceased. A hysterectomy was advised. The necessity of the surgery raised another problem for me. What would I do with my three little ones? Mom was one possibility.

After my father died, my mother had to sell the house, and she landed a job at Coe Manufacturing where she met a wonderful man named Ray Nute. His two previous marriages had ended in divorce, and that was of concern to us. Mom proved wiser than we. She was determined to wait a year after my father's death, and so one year and one month after my father died, they were married in a simple service. Our fears for her were groundless. Mom spent nearly twenty happy years with her new husband.

With the surgery, I needed her help. When I called her to ask her to watch the kid's, she said no. I was crushed. What was I going to do? There was no one else. I even offered to pay her. She wouldn't budge. In a few days, she relented and agreed to come.

As my pregnancy progressed, I mused about the birth of Liz, my sister Linda's daughter. After the delivery, in nineteen sixty-six, my mom came down to Cuyahoga Falls and stayed a full week with her. That cut me like a knife. When I desperately needed her help, she grudgingly came for two days after considerable begging on my part. The reason was obvious. After all these years, I was still the outsider. Linda was the true daughter, and I was the worthless one. I never felt it more acutely than I did then. The scar on my heart remains to this day.

The surgery was uneventful, and I came home from the hospital on time. Mom stayed two more days, then left. I was barely ambulatory.

Kids and ED

Art helped all he could when he was home, but mostly, I was on my own during the long day.

Somehow, I got through the convalescence. Then, my monster poked his head from his hole. What did I expect? I wasn't worth her time or the trouble. I never had been. Why should I think I was now? Just because I proved I could have a few kids didn't make me worth anything. One of these days, I'd admit that to myself and stop expecting things from other people. With a sigh, I accepted my victim's role and settled into motherhood with the attitude of servant to husband and children.

At this point in my life, what had been a periodic exercise at weight control became a true way of life. Propelled by the stress and responsibilities of children ages seven, five, and one, and the desire to be the perfect wife, I restricted food in earnest. I might be less than successful at my other jobs, but I was as in control of my diet as a pilot landing a passenger jet. No way would I end up a middle-aged, chubby she-creature. In no time at all, I was down to a hundred pounds.

CHAPTER 8

Running Through the Years

Those of us with ED are running away from something; our childhood; our situation; our mate, or most of the times, ourselves. It helps us sharpen our obsessive-compulsive behaviors that are inherent in all anorexics. The next decade of my life became the brutal training ground for that behavior as I ran away from myself.

The only words appropriate for this time are, "busy little girl." The busier I was, the happier I was. Since this was the decade that ED took complete control of my life, I will add "sick little girl," to these ten years.

Eating disorders are symptoms of a greater, complex underlying problem. All my life, I handled the stresses of life in a pathologic way. My vision was distorted by the constant need to prove myself; do more; accomplish more; serve more to earn the love and respect of my family and friends. That defect, coupled with an inadequate personality, set me up for ED's takeover of my life. I could never do enough; accomplish enough; serve enough in my own eyes to accomplish my desired goal. In the end, the only thing I could control was what I ate.

This was also the decade that my perception of the world around me, and my relationship with others warped like a wet piece of plywood.

My interpretation of what others were telling me became fuel for the fire of my inadequacy. Since I couldn't control what I thought others were telling me, I went back to the only thing I could control, and ED loved it.

I also had no idea how to make myself happy. I didn't like myself, and if I didn't like me, surely no one else could like me either. I refined the use of others emotions to replace my own. If I thought Art wasn't happy, I wasn't happy. If the children didn't seem happy, I wasn't happy. That's not a great way to live, but I didn't know any other way.

In short, I customized my lifestyle to fit my disease perfectly. I have always been an early riser. I was up at the crack of dawn to get a running start on the day. My first task was to make myself a strong pot of coffee. The caffeine was necessary to jump start my nutritionally starved system.

Next came breakfast for my husband and three hungry children. And, there were lunches to pack. With all that work and a time schedule to meet, I certainly didn't have time to eat. When the refuse of breakfast had been cleared away, the dishes were in the dishwasher and the gang was off to work or school, I treated myself to a second cup of coffee.

During the summer, or on weekends when everyone was home, lunchtime was a carbon copy of breakfast with the equivalent consumption of coffee. If nobody was there for lunch, I busied myself with cleaning, a craft project, or ran errands to avoid eating.

By the time dinner rolled around, I was wired from the caffeine and hungrier than a she-bear after hibernation. If I could keep my intake of food to the five or six hundred calorie range, I didn't purge. If I couldn't, I did my magic trick and solved the problem. I lived in a house of plenty, and for forty years I consumed no more calories than a concentration camp prisoner.

Perversely, when we went out to dinner, I seldom purged. I restricted my meals to salads with no dressing, broiled fish or scallop dishes without sauce, or boiled shrimp. I was proud of myself for being in such good control.

Discovering the Monster Within

Like any young family, the major thrust of this period involved raising the children. Art's job required significant amounts of travel. So, much of the time, the children were my responsibility. That suited me fine. The busy little girl had more to do and less time to think about eating.

Because Art had to be gone so much, I tried to make things about his trips special for the children. I would take them with me to pick him up at the airport. We'd go early and watch the planes from the observation deck. I cooked special meals and tried to make each homecoming a mini celebration. Of course I was careful not to allow any resentment to surface. Nobody liked resentful people, and I was hard enough to like already.

What did I resent? I knew Art had no choice about the travel. One part of me needed the extra work to keep busy. Another part resented being in the position of constant disciplinarian. I was always the bad guy who put the damper on everything. He went places, saw things and came home the good guy. When he was home, the discipline still remained my duty. Naturally, the kid's were more eager to please him than me, and it grated on me. I did the dirty work, and he got the glory. That angered me. Behind my back, the kids called me, 'the Bitch!'

When I told Art about the uncomplimentary title, he said, "You probably deserved it."

He can't remember that exchange, but it's ingrained in my memory. Because my perception of the world was so different then, he could be right. Did the conversation actually occur, or did I make the assumption it was his answer from some insignificant comment he made? I don't know the truth, but I am so convinced it happened, I could pass a lie detector test if asked about it. Did Art block out the unkind response? I don't know. But he would line up behind me at the same machine, take the lie detector test and pass. The mind is a powerful and frightening thing, particularly when its vision of the world is clouded.

Lacking the communication skills to express my feelings, I couldn't talk to him about it, then. With no concept of how to manage my anger and resentment other than punishing myself, that's what I did.

Despite my problems, I am a good cook. My friend, who has had some training as a gourmet chef told me that he was amazed that I could cook so many delicious things and prepare scrumptious desserts without every tasting anything myself. I always felt it was my job to cook. I loved to do it, and at times tried to force feed my family, another trait many of us with ED regularly exhibit. Mom had never liked to cook, and it showed. I was determined to be better at it than she was.

Each of my children picked a decade to be a problem for me. In the seventies it was David. Although my personality might be described as energetic, I had no previous contact with a truly hyperactive person until my son came along. I didn't handle it well at first.

There was a public park behind our house on Bancroft Street, and I liked to treat the children to a trip to the park. David was only nine months old, and still in the crawling stage when, I took my little brood there for a summer afternoon of play.

My first task was to find a shady spot next to the swings and sandbox where I could sit in comfort to watch them. That accomplished, I put David in the sandbox with his plastic bucket and shovel. I turned my back on him long enough to buckle Carolyn into the kiddy swing. Turning around, to my horror, the sandbox was empty!

Frantically I swept the park with my eyes. We had been alone when we came in. No stranger had been near enough to snatch him. Bizarre thoughts of alien abduction filled my head when I heard a giggle from the direction of the older children's play area. From the top of the gigantic sliding board, David smiled down at me with his little crooked grin. As far as I know, this was the first time he walked in his life, but there he was ten feet in the air. The sight took years off my life. I was so panic stricken that I'm still not sure how I got him down.

On another occasion, I went down to the basement to transfer the washing to the dryer. Just as I finished my chore, the phone rang.

Dashing up the stairs I snatched the handset from the cradle. It was my next-door neighbor, Helen Moore.

"Pat, do you know that David is out back walking on top of the fence?" she asked.

"I just saw him through the window."

A six feet high, wooden privacy fence separated our back yard from Helen's. There was David, walking the flat cap rail like one of the Flying Walendas! I had no idea he knew how to open a door. He had to stand on tiptoe just to reach the knob. We brought him safely to terra firma, and I thanked Helen profusely.

I soon learned with his activity level I couldn't leave him alone for a minute. Safety precautions with doors, windows, medicine cabinets and bottle tops became a daily routine.

Despite my best efforts, he still outwitted me on occasion. One afternoon, when I was certain he was in his room, I went upstairs to see what he was doing. He was gone! I found him across the street, sitting on my neighbor's curb. Fortunately, our dead end street kept the traffic sparse. Those vehicles venturing to the end of the street were almost always neighbors, well aware of the rug-rat infestation of our street.

Investigating the incident, I found that at age ten months, David could vault over the side of his crib with such ease that it astounded me. We added six inch high extension rails to the sides of the crib, but the learning curve to surmount the added height was less than a week. A crib net was next, but it just entangled him, so he won. We moved him to a twin bed. Once we found him sleeping under the bed. David would simply go until he dropped. At dinner one evening, he fell asleep while eating and ended up face-first in his mashed potatoes.

Although I never attended a religious school, I was as guilt ridden as any Catholic school girl. Since everything in the world revolved around me, another common anorexic symptom, I was convinced everything was my fault. It was a *prima-fascia* reason to feel guilty. In David's case, the guilt was over the time it was taking me to keep him out of mischief. It meant I was neglecting Carolyn and later, Calvin.

Running Through the Years

We always tried to make the children's birthdays special. Art always took the birthday child out to dinner alone, while I did something special with the other two. When the guest of honor arrived back home, the whole family celebrated with cake and ice cream. Of course, I was so busy arranging everything that I didn't have time to eat the goodies, but I always joined the celebration.

Carolyn went to nursery school three days per week. They weren't as sophisticated then as they are today, but rudimentary skills were still taught. It became readily apparent that she had a mild problem with dyslexia. Waves of guilt threatened to drown me. Had I caused it? Did my eating habits damage my child? We arranged for her to visit a child psychologist, and the twenty minute trips each way to the appointments gave me time to be alone with Carolyn and focus only on her. It eased my guilt feelings about the attention David required, but in the end I wonder if it had any effect on her at all.

Calvin had physical problems as well. Before he was even a year of age, he was diagnosed with bilateral inguinal hernias and had to have surgery. He came through it with flying colors.

David was assaulted by numerous allergies, and ear infections tormented the hapless child. Art and I tried to recount the number of times tubes had to be inserted in his ears on an emergency basis, and we honestly couldn't remember. I had a standing appointment at the ENT office. Dr. Milo told his staff that when I called, David was to receive an immediate appointment because he was in trouble. Dr. Milo is a dear sweet man with no sense of time whatsoever. On good days he would be an hour behind. Imagine how long walk-ins had to wait!

My two edged sword cleaved the air. I felt quite noble for patiently waiting hour upon hour with my sick child and simultaneously guilt ridden about neglecting the other two. In the back of my mind, I wondered if in some way my eating behavior had damaged this child, too. Instead of confronting the eating disorder and changing my behavior, I asked ED to sooth my guilt and lower my tension levels.

Discovering the Monster Within

Following David's surgeries, he had to be kept quiet. With a child who was never still for a nanosecond, that was a chore. We had a sleeper sofa in the living room, and I found that if I opened it, David would lie there with me for a little while. Other diversions were necessary for longer stays, so I played records and read countless books to him.

I found out later how much Carolyn truly resented her siblings, particularly the time I spent with David. Years after David no longer required the attention; she threw it up to me.

"You never pulled out the sofa and read to me," she said accusingly.

At the time, her words felt like daggers in my heart. Again, everything was about me … me … me and my inadequacies. I never stopped to put things, like Carolyn's selfishness, into the equation. It was too easy to blame myself. After all, I was worthless anyhow.

Our old neighbors, Ed and Eldora Thorn lived in Chicago at the time. Ed had a degree in speech and rhetoric and was teaching in a college. We decided to take Calvin there to be baptized. It had been a long time between vacations, and we felt we deserved one. It was a wonderful visit, and we were the proudest of parents as our little boy received the holy sacrament of baptism.

Then whoosh! The two-edged sword cleaved my happiness. On the way home, all three children broke out in chicken-pox! By the time we reached Akron, the car resembled a pediatric ward.

Carolyn was taking ballet lessons at the time. She was too sick to perform in the final recital. I felt so bad for her, but she put her tutu to good use. Several weeks later, she dressed David up in her recital tutu! Since he broke out with the pox first, I think she blamed him for her misery. It was a big-sister's cruel revenge, although David never appreciated it.

Aside from their illnesses, the children were a great outlet for my busy little girl persona. They all took piano lessons and later on a second instrument. Art is an accomplished musician specializing in trombone. Except for my off key singing, I possessed no musical aptitude at all.

Inadequate again! I made up for my inadequacies by hauling everyone to their lessons and overseeing practice sessions.

Next, scouts occupied my time; Cub Scouts; Brownie Scouts; Girl and Boy Scouts. Adding t-ball, soccer, basketball, school band, art and swimming classes, plus anything else that struck their fancy, put me on a transportation and scheduling merry-go-round. We did them all, and the more we did, the more I felt I had to do. My reward for my servitude was an excuse not to eat. I was too busy. I'd eat after the activity of the moment, but I never did.

It wasn't all work with the children. We had fun too. With three of them and a budget, we did a lot of family camping. We had a small camping trailer and spent many glorious weekends at a campground not far from home. Cal followed Art around like a puppy dog as we set up camp. Cal always was a visual learner, and his keen observations allowed him to pick up many skills, such as woodworking and electrical work, simply by watching others.

When we camped, it was very difficult to purge, so I used my sharpened restricting techniques. It was easy to stay busy at the campsite. As long as I had plenty of chores, I didn't have to bother eating.

There is an image in my mind from those camping trips that epitomizes my family. Art and Calvin, the inveterate campers, fussed with roasting the hotdogs over the fire. Carolyn sat alone on a large rock, daydreaming, while David ran in circles around the camp for no apparent reason. I'll always love that old camp site, that's probably a housing development, now. The only constant in life is change.

Besides being home room mother for all three children and volunteering for everything and anything from band activities to P. T. A. drives, I kept my plate full with domestic activities. I made most of the children's clothes, as well as my own. I had two gardens, made the curtains and drapes for the house and fell in love with needle point. At times, I got up in the middle of the night to work on my latest needle point project. Many of us with ED use excessive exercise to burn off offending calories. It wasn't my conscious purpose, but it worked anyhow.

Discovering the Monster Within

A classic example of the behavior was a weekend campout with Carolyn's scout troop. I shopped, planned the meals, arranged the transportation, and was constantly on the phone with the parents and the girls. Delegate? What's delegate? I had to supervise *everything* to be certain the weekend was perfect for each and every girl. I skipped meals, and no one noticed. I doubt that I consumed a thousand calories the entire weekend. I was a happy camper and so was E.D.

I was driven to do, do, do. There was a sense of accomplishment with each completed task that lasted only a heartbeat until it was replaced with the uncontrollable urge to do more. I had to prove my worth to my family, my friends and my neighbors, just as I had to do in the Archer family. No matter what I did, it was never enough.

The other thing I wondered about was where I got the energy to do it all. It certainly didn't come from the food I ate. Perhaps David's hyperactivity was inherited from me. Even if it wasn't, my personality let me take the blame.

My family observed my eating habits, but no one accused me of anything. I feel sure both mothers were suspicious. My mom confronted me directly about it. Of course I lied. Art's mom actually followed me to the bathroom to see if I was purging. They never caught me at anything. I was too polished an anorexic for that, but it wouldn't have mattered if they did. I wasn't ready for help yet.

During this time, my relationship with my brother, Dave, who was studying for the ministry, was strained to the breaking point. He seldom communicated with any of us. When he was invited to visit us, his answer was always the same. He told us his church was his family, and they needed him more than we did.

I took it personally, because I had felt it was me that he hated. But, he acted the same way toward all of us. It hurt us all, but it crushed, Mom. She idolized him, and never could understand why he refused the Godly command to honor his mother.

We loved his children, and still do. Although he seemed to care nothing for our children, we never missed one of his children's graduations. He lived in New York and Pennsylvania during this time and claimed he had neither the time nor inclination to visit relatives he couldn't tolerate anyhow.

Dave's constant rejection, criticism and holier-than-thou attitude turned my hurt to anger. At first, Art tried to understand him and to accept his strange behavior. After awhile, he quit trying. When he saw how much Dave's attitude hurt me, he began to dislike Dave. It took my sisters and me decades to finally realized it was Dave's problem and his loss, not ours. My poor mom never did see it. It broke her heart. I kept praying that one day we could work things out.

In nineteen seventy-three, tragedy struck our family, and the devastation it left in its wake tainted lives for the next two decades. Bob, my sister Beverly's husband, shot himself to death, leaving Beverly with three young children and no means of support.

I was stunned and unable to believe he had done such a thing. At the same time, I was angry with Bob for doing such a stupid thing to my sister. What was she going to do? Why had he done it? Who was to blame? There must have been warning signs, but none of us saw them. Was there some way I could have prevented it from happening? Could Art, or one of my children, do the same thing?

Bob left no suicide note, so none of my questions were ever answered. Bob's family must have blamed Beverly, because they quickly extracted themselves from her life, and worst of all from the children's lives. I so wanted to fix things for Beverly, but I couldn't. One more time, I wasn't up to the task.

Whenever I could, I had Bev's three kids down to visit. ED relished those weekends, because I was so busy I couldn't possibly have time to eat. One morning, the kids had come to the kitchen for breakfast, and I asked them what they wanted to eat. I had a plethora of breakfast treats like eggs, bacon, waffles, hot cakes, sausage and cereal.

Looking at me askance, Bev said, "Are you crazy? Don't ask them, just feed them."

Discovering the Monster Within

Beverly didn't understand. I always had to fix everything for everybody. My only joy was the joy of others. If the kids were happy, I could be happy. I couldn't help myself. Each child had to have what I never had. If there was a need, a want, whatever it was, I tried to give it to them. It was as if by giving them what I never had, I could retrospectively deal with my childhood privation. Life is not about making up for the past. It is about understanding the past and refusing to allow it to adversely affect the future. It took me nearly a lifetime to figure that out.

I continued to do what I could for Beverly. Art tolerated the situation, and tried to understand. She got a job and raised the children as best she could. My sister became a slovenly housekeeper, and began to gain even more weight making the situation a lot tougher.

Cancer reared its ugly head in the family again in this decade. Art's dad was diagnosed with prostate cancer. PSA testing wasn't in vogue yet, and the disease crept up on unsuspecting men in the prime of their maturity. By the time it was diagnosed, it was too late for a cure.

His symptoms began as vague neurological signs progressing rapidly to paralysis. An emergency surgery was performed to decompress his cancer riddled spine. He was started on Estrogen therapy, since modern anti-androgens were still a decade away. Radiation therapy was added to the larger patches of cancer in the bone. My heart ached as I watched this vital man lying there in that bed.

Dad Burkley tackled his cancer as he did everything else in his life. He fought it like the demon it was. He made it to a wheelchair. Through months of therapy, he progressed from the chair to a walker and finally to a three point cane. The rest of his life was clouded with pain, but he never gave up. His cancer went into remission, and he was able to be with us fifteen more years.

Our relationship with my family was even more strained. We never spent a great deal of time with my family. Ray, mom's new husband, was wonderful to her, and loved her as my father never could. They spent more time with Linda, Dan and Beverly, further cementing the concept that I was the unworthy, unwanted daughter. In truth, it was as much my fault as theirs.

Art had little to nothing in common with my family. He didn't fish, enjoy primitive camping with three small kids, gardening, or antique collecting and restoring. He found the "casual," housekeeping of my family and their greasy meals not to his liking. So, we spent more time with his folks. Since his father was so ill, I didn't mind. Besides, Dad Burkley always seemed genuinely happy to see me.

Now, I wish I had been more insistent. They were my family, after all. I loved them and wanted to be a bigger part of their lives. I never considered talking to Art about anything, or actually asking him how he felt. It was easier for Ms. Victim to assume that we didn't visit my family because he didn't want to.

In reality, Art's mom and Dad visited our home frequently, while we had to drive several hours each way to visit my parents. I ignored that and interpreted every situation in a way that put me, the victim, at the epicenter. How wasteful.

Unfortunately, Beverly's decline reinforced his position. I handled my problems by denial, internalization and bulimia. Beverly handled hers by a decent into slovenliness.

Besides taking Bev's children from time to time, we also cleaned her house periodically. On one horrid occasion we found cooking pots covered with mold and mounds of smelly dishes in the sink. There was so much dirt and garbage in the carpet that potatoes actually sprouted from the detritus. When I changed one of the children's beds, I removed a shabby set of brown bed sheets. After I washed them, they were filthy white ones. I felt pity and sorrow, while Art felt revulsion. I couldn't blame him. Although I had caused none of it, I felt deeply ashamed of my sister and personalized it as my own.

We didn't have a large cadre of friends in those days. Art didn't seem to cultivate many friendships at work. Though I never asked, I assumed it was due to me. He had to be ashamed of me. I was plump, unattractive, and not intelligent enough to mingle with his friends.

Discovering the Monster Within

Convincing myself that all these ludicrous ideas were, I accepted my plight.

My perception of life was so out of proportion, I never saw the truth. In fact, the company had regular parties that we attended. Art didn't socialize with fellow workers because he was their boss and didn't feel comfortable socializing in a way that could create a conflict of interest. I never even considered that. The situation had to be about me, didn't it?

In the early seventies, we met three other couples who would play profound roles in our lives. Although I didn't realize it at the time, they would be counted as life long friends. It has taken me three decades to understand how they felt about me. I always assumed they were friends because of Art. I had to completely change the way I interpreted the things I saw and heard before I could understand that they were friends of *mine*, too.

I met Jan Porter one day when I was signing Carolyn up for an art class. Jan was there with her daughter, Karen. Carolyn and Karen began gabbing like old friends, and we found they went to the same school, and that we lived in the same neighborhood. She introduced me to her friend, Nancy Roberts. Around the same time, I met my new neighbor, Pat Summers, who had moved in two doors down.

We all had a common interest, bridge, and decided that a monthly, rotational, Saturday night bridge and dinner group might be fun. Imagine, me getting excited over dinner. Dick Porter, Bob Roberts and Jack Summers, the respective husbands, agreed. It was an instant hit. For the next twenty plus years, we seldom missed a monthly meeting, even after everyone else left the old neighborhood.

Despite being their equal, they intimidated me. None of them ever did anything to deserve that title; it was just my inadequacy. Since everyone had different backgrounds and occupations, we never talked shop, but everything else was fair game. I learned some of my best jokes on Saturday nights, even though Art had to explain one or two of them to me.

Running Through the Years

The other women were self-assured and intellectual, with broad general backgrounds. They were partners with their men, and not afraid to debate or disagree with them. They couldn't relate to my dependence on and deference to Art. My insecurity wouldn't let me express an opinion on current events or politics, even though I had them. My new friends realized something I didn't. They saw my intellect and ability and assumed that I chose not to be involved in things because I didn't care. Still, these Saturday nights were some of the happiest of my life.

True to ED, I remember the first bridge and dinner because it was at my house. I made ham and scalloped potatoes. Why? Because I knew I would have to eat, and this meal was the easiest one to purge!

Over the years, the other couples drifted away from the neighborhood to bigger houses, new neighborhoods and other school systems. Since none of them were more than twenty minutes away, we remained close friends and continued our monthly bacchanals. These were my friends, and I was very happy for them. Yet, their success merely emphasized my inadequacy, and I punished myself for it. None of them has ever said a purposely hurtful thing to me, but I had a way of taking even their most benign comment and using it as a whip to flagellate myself with.

My perception of my world remained flawed, and I continued to function under the premise that the more I did, the more I accomplished, the more I would be accepted. Strange as it seems, I was simultaneously paralyzed by indecision. I never picked furniture, drapery material or wallpaper by myself. I couldn't make up my mind. It was so important for me to please others, I was afraid I wouldn't make the proper choice. It even came down to what dress I should wear. I constantly needed reinforcement from others. I still do. If I want something that Art doesn't, and I get it, it doesn't make me happy. But, I'm working on that.

Over time, I began to resent Art's control over me. I had given it to him and still didn't have the courage to make my own decisions, but I became irrationally angry about his control over my life. I stewed about it while ED cheered.

Discovering the Monster Within

I was so wrapped up in myself, that I never realized that Art had issues of his own. He felt that *things* were important. While I was growing up, I never had any things of value, so they were not important to me. In Art's family, things were quite different.

Art's family moved frequently. Each move involved redecoration. Sometimes, his mother redecorated for no reason at all. One day, Art's dad came home from work to find she had given away the dining room table. Things were always in a state of flux.

For balance, Art needed a stable environment. That was one of the reasons we never seriously considered moving from our Bancroft Street home as our friends had done. Sameness was Art's life preserver. When he felt the urge to change, it was always in a small way. Repaper a room here; paint a wall there.

Ignorant of his motivation, each time he did something, I was positive the reason was me. I didn't help him do it right in the first place. It had to be the result of my bad judgment. As each project granted Art solace, it filled me with self-loathing for my inadequacy. When that loathing was internalized, it became anger. I was rapidly becoming a very angry woman with no concept of how to express that anger.

At this time, two major things happened that would effect the next two decades. In September of nineteen seventy-nine, I took a three month refresher course in nursing, and started back to work at a local Osteopathic Hospital, and Art suffered his first severe bout of depression.

I was so busy diving into my victim well that I had no clue how deep it really was. I blithely continued to dote on the children; please Art everyway I could think of; read cookbooks as though they were Gospel; crank out needlepoint like a machine; eat and purge.

CHAPTER 9

Descent into Purgatory

Many anorexics are so consumed by their disease that they stop everything else in their lives to concentrate on feeding their individual species of the monster. I never experienced that aspect of the disease. It gradually consumed me, like a slow growing cancer. The next two decades of my life were a gradual descent into the bowels of a nightmare.

I was working the three to eleven shift at the hospital, and the routine was comforting. Get the kids off to school after feeding them a nourishing breakfast. Be certain no one forgot anything essential to a day at public school, as they hurried out the door. With so many important items on my agenda, there was no time for food, but I continued to try to drown myself with coffee.

When they were gone, I sipped coffee and perused the morning newspaper. Though I never realized it, my energy reserves were dangerously low, and I needed to sit for a time to recharge my batteries. I lied to myself. I was only enjoying a few moments of selfish pleasure that I richly deserved for being so good to my family.

Respite over, it was time for action again. There were beds to be made, floors to be swept or mopped and laundry to be done. Thank

God I was too busy to eat. Another cup of coffee was always nice. A second pot was frequently necessary.

In the afternoon, I fixed dinner. Just because I was working, it didn't mean I was free to shirk my domestic responsibilities. I had to give, give, give. It was the only way I could mean anything to my family.

Around one o'clock, I began my own gorge fest. For an hour, I crammed myself with spaghetti, mashed potatoes, and bread, anything that would come back easily. I ate until I was stuffed, in classic bulimic fashion. Before leaving for work, I performed my magic trick for ED, and up it came in all its partially digested glory, along with more enamel from my teeth. ED never failed to give me a standing ovation.

I suppose I was fortunate enough to retain enough nutrition from the food while I allowed it to remain in my system to keep me from starving to death. It cured my hunger. I never had to go to dinner at work. I was pleased with myself. I was in control, and it was all *about control.*

At work I made friends with Mary Jane, a jovial giant of a woman. We formed the classic odd couple. At six feet and nearly three hundred pounds, she was Jeff to my Mutt.

We made a great nursing team. Each of us did what the other couldn't stand to do. Bowel content were anathema to me, while Mary Jane gagged at the thought of mucous. Each of us helped with the others phobia. It was awesome.

Mary Jane accepted my thinness, and I accepted her obesity. But, in my mind, I felt as obese as she was. ED does that to you. Aside from occasional friendly teasing, it was never an issue. Others in my life accepted me, but I couldn't see it. With Mary Jane, I could. Why? I have no idea.

The only real bone of contention between us was my dependency on Art. She simply could not understand it. She would always begin her 'constructive criticism' with her patented irreverent phrase.

She would say "Piss on that shit, Pat! You don't need any man to tell you what to do. You have a brain girl. You have a job. Use your head.

Get some backbone." Perhaps this kind of attitude was part of the reason that Art never could understand our friendship.

For the three years I worked at the hospital, no one ever saw me eat. A cup of coffee at the nurses' lounge was all I allowed myself. To go to dinner with my colleagues was too dangerous. They accepted me as an equal, and I might be caught up in the spirit of the moment. I might succumb to a bite of real food. If I took a bite of the forbidden fruit, I might find it as sweet as Eve did, and I would be lost.

The behavior held for the shop picnic for the night shift nurses I hosted in my backyard. I never took a bite of anything. How could I? There was so much to do; so much to oversee that I couldn't possibly have time to eat.

Because I had to leave for work before Art came home, we purchased a second car, a stick shift, nineteen seventy-nine Chevrolet. I was happy to have my own car, but ED wouldn't let me completely enjoy it. He quickly reminded me I didn't deserve it.

The car was the source of one special memory for me. One night in winter, a lake effect snowstorm, that rarely wanders as far south as Akron, roared down on us like a runaway freight train from Lake Erie. Ice and snow spun a cocoon of white around our community. Trudging to the parking lot, I dreaded standing in the cold wind scraping the ice from my car. The cold still bothers me as much as it did when I was a child.

To my surprise and delight, my car was clean. The windows were scraped down to clean glass and the snow had been lovingly brushed away by my wonderful husband. Art had driven the five miles from home to clean my car for me. After such an act of kindness and love, why couldn't I understand that I had worth in Art's eyes? Blinded by ED, I simply couldn't.

My job at the hospital was part time, so I found things to occupy my free time. Jack, my neighbor from the bridge group called me one day. He was chairman of the local medical college department of urology.

His office nurse had just died, and he asked me if I could fill in until he found a replacement.

I was delighted, honored and frightened all at the same time. Through my own insecurity, and my old school nurse's training that deified physicians, I had placed Jack on a pedestal. What if I couldn't do it? What if it didn't work out? With my heart in my mouth I accepted his invitation to work for him.

Jack had office hours three half-days a week. Two were mornings and one an afternoon. It was perfect for me. I could work nights, and handle Jack's office in the day. I didn't work at the hospital on Thursday so I could see patients with him in the afternoon. Great! There were more things for me to do and less time to eat.

Working with Jack was a high. I quickly learned the special nursing skills required in urology. I took charge of the office with gusto. At work, I was *in control*. I am a good nurse, though I can only recently admit that to myself. And, I proved it every time I put on my starched white nurse's cap. We wore those caps as badges of honor in my day. I think the profession has lost something by doing away with them.

In time, Jack found a full time nurse, which in truth he needed. As I left his office, it was with mixed emotions. Wasn't I good enough to be offered the full time job? Had I done something wrong? Again, rejection reared its head. Though I never showed it, it hurt.

Jack remains one of my oldest and dearest friends. He made a wise decision before he asked me to work for him. Valuing my friendship above all else, he wanted nothing to jeopardize that. What if some office issue forced him to let me go? If things didn't work out, what would happen if he had to fire me? Unwilling to risk that, Jack talked it over with his wife, Pat, and they agreed my employment should only be temporary.

Jack has subsequently told me that his only regret was not sharing his thinking with me until many years later. We agree that we could probably have worked well together for our entire careers with no problems. We also agree that Jack's choice was a wise one.

Descent into Purgatory

Eventually, I had to admit that the evening shift interfered with too many of the children's activities. Carolyn went to her first prom, and I was at work. ED said, "Bad Mom!" The kids were in band and musical performances, and I had to work. ED said, "Bad Mom!" Taking a fifty percent pay cut, I went to work for a local urgent care center. At least it was a nine to four job.

ED wasn't pleased with this change of pace. I found I couldn't go all day without some form of nourishment. Since I had no store of reserves, as the day wore on, I became dangerously fatigued. I needed some form of nourishment.

My remedies for the situation were ludicrous. I took a mushroom or two to work with me. Imitating a psychotic bunny, I nibbled on them all day long. Trim was the name of a ghastly-tasting, instant soup containing ten calories per serving that was popular with the dieters of the period. I mixed it with three times the amount of water required and sipped the vile broth as if it were lobster bisque. At supper, I added three or four hundred calories more.

That year, Calvin entered puberty and declared war on Art and me. At first, we wrote it off to junior high jitters. He progressively became mouthy, disobedient, disrespectful and slovenly.

In the summer, Calvin climbed on a roof supposedly to retrieve an errant Frisby. Jumping from the roof, he broke his knuckle. Our local hand surgeon had to pin it. He started junior high in a cast. We made countless trips to the doctor and the therapist. It was great for me. I could be the good mother and try to atone for not protecting my son from himself. Cal refused to cooperate with the therapy and carries a permanently crooked finger as his reward. Punishing myself, I avoided food. Like a concentration camp prisoner, I worked from dawn till dark while subsisting on less than the nine hundred calories in a starvation diet.

Calvin sought out wild companions and began to drink, carouse and smoke. Who was to blame for his waywardness? Me of course! It's hard to believe anyone could be as self-centered as I was. If I didn't push the earth, it wouldn't turn. If anything happened anywhere on the surface of that planet, it was somehow connected to me and some unknown sin I had knowingly or unknowingly committed. Since I was telling God he had made a mistake with my appearance, I might as well just take some of His authority away from Him, too.

David gave us a scare that fall. On Thursday after school, the high school band practiced their Friday football halftime routine under the lights at the stadium. After the drill, a rough and tumble football game frequently broke out among the band members.

Imagine my shock and horror as a gurney burst through the door of the urgent care center where I was working with my son strapped to it! He was having chest pain and trouble breathing. David had fallen during the game, and a much larger boy had fallen on David's chest, crushing his rib cage. Frightened and in pain, he had insisted on being taken to where his mother worked.

Fortunately, the final damage was a sprain of the joints where the ribs attach to the breast bone and a mild bruise of his heart. No permanent damage. An unfortunate accident caused by adolescent horseplay? Of course it wasn't. I hadn't properly supervised my child. I was working too much. I should have been there to pick him up after band practice. I, I, I, it was all I could think of. "Atta girl," ED whispered.

That spring, Carolyn graduated from high school. Of my three children, Carolyn was the one I could never get close too. Always aloof, she became truly distant this summer. Preparing to attend college in the fall, she worked and kept to herself most of the time. I was so intent on my other problems, I didn't recognize the danger this gulf between us, that rapidly became a chasm, represented.

When school restarted in the fall, Calvin's rebellion escalated to civil war. David, involved in everything, required a full-time chauffeur. Carolyn, now at college, joined The Campus Crusade For Christ, a decision that would eventually wreck havoc with my family. As for me, I starved my way through the rest of the year.

Two years later, David left for college. It was important for him to live on campus and enjoy the complete college experience although he could have commuted the twenty minute drive to the University of Akron Campus. We helped him pack and bundled him off to his apartment. I had no idea how traumatic it was for him.

David told me that he sat down in his room and looked around. He didn't know anybody, and felt totally alone. What if something happened to me, he had wondered? How long before anyone would know? Would anyone even care?

Immediately, I accepted full responsibility for my child's normal separation anxiety. I was not a good mother. Where was I when he needed me? Why hadn't I prepared him for life on his own? Why didn't he feel more loved and secure? More excuses to punish myself. ED was so happy.

Once, I truly was guilty of neglecting my son. While playing a pickup game of basketball, David lacerated his head. He called home, and after a few questions, I determined the cut wasn't that bad. David could be excitable. Besides, I had just plated dinner for the rest of the family.

Following dinner, I took time for my magic act before departing for David's apartment. When I saw the laceration, I took him straight to the emergency room. Fifteen stitches later, I was so guilt ridden that I wanted to crawl under a rock. With my guilt levels so high, the only way I knew to relieve them was by initiating the binge-purge cycle.

Consumed by her commitment to Campus Crusade for Christ, Carolyn decided not to return home that summer. Instead, she went to Madison, Wisconsin to continue her Christian mission. I thought that peculiar. Didn't missionaries go to Africa or China?

Art and I went to visit her and took a day trip to the Wisconsin Dells. It was the last time I ever talked to a loving daughter who had any regard for me as a person.

After dinner one evening, the two of us walked along a tree shaded pathway. The moat between us seemed to shrink. She told me that she had been called by God to travel behind the Iron Curtain. God would take care of her, and I shouldn't worry. If anything happened, she didn't want me to grieve, because she would be doing God's will. I started to protest, but thought better of it, and asked the questions any concerned parent would ask when faced with such a declaration from an only daughter.

She answered them with a sweet serenity. Then, she told me I was a child of God and that God loved me, too. In time, I should be proud of that and love myself in return. Her words caused a curtain, heavier than the Iron One she was to cross, to close between us.

My diseased ears heard the most unbelievable thing imaginable. God, love me? Nothing about me was loveable. It was not possible. I wasn't worthy of God's love. My brother, Dave, reminded me of the same thing once when he tried to discuss God's place in my life with me, and I told him I wasn't about to give up control of my life to God. Control was that critical to me.

Carolyn got a different message from my words. I suspect that she thought I was rejecting God and demeaning her work. I may never know. We never talked about it. She crossed back to her side of the void and rowed further away from me. The closer she moved to her vision of God, the more it blinded her to her mother's love. Lacking the persistence of the Christ she served, she never tried to talk to me about God again.

Of course she was right. God did love me, but I was in no condition to realize it then. I lacked the self esteem to even believe that it was possible. Thank God I have found Him, and He has allowed me to see that worth. Unfortunately, my pitiful state that beautiful day in Wisconsin may have cost me my child.

That whole episode seems so foolish to me now. We were a religious family. Art and I belonged to the First Methodist Church of Cuyahoga Falls before we had children. I was active in the women's groups and actually helped found the Rebecca Circle there. One summer, I even taught a Bible study. We took all the kids to church and Sunday school; they sang in the church vocal groups and went to summer camp.

Descent into Purgatory

Unfortunately, we severed our relationship with that congregation when they refused to print in the bulletin that Carolyn had joined the Campus Crusade for Christ. In retrospect, I see why, but then we could only perceive it as an unchristian snub from the church that helped shape her faith. In time, we found another place to worship.

I have frequently asked myself how I could go to church on a regular basis since I was a teenager, and never understand God's love and compassion. Why did it take me half-a-century to understand it? I have always had a strong faith, but unfortunately for Art, he lost some of his. Carolyn's subsequent actions, and the attitude of my brother, Dave, caused Art to doubt his Christian principles. Fortunately, God is working with Art to heal those painful wounds, and he is back in church with me again.

That same year, after discovering he had been sneaking out at night, we took Calvin to a counselor. We left the office in disbelief when he told us, "Let him get in trouble while he's still a minor so he won't have a record as an adult." Frustrated, and wanting to help our child, not acquiesce to a police record, we transformed the house into a virtual holding cell, and thought we had all forms of egress barred.

Undeterred, Calvin tried to sneak out of the house after hours for a clandestine meeting with his drinking buddies. His only escape was through his bedroom window. When he jumped to the ground from the second story, he cracked the vertebra in his back. A trip to the emergency room ended in a back brace and a prescription for physical therapy.

Calvin had a paper route, so Art and I took over that chore while Calvin imitated a turtle. I remember Carolyn washing his hair when she was home from college while he whined about soap in his eyes. Thank God he healed without permanent damage.

Eventually, David and Carolyn both went back to college leaving Calvin alone with the enemy! We tried our level best. We never left him alone, ferrying him to and from each activity. The more we did, the angrier he became, and the more I blamed myself for everything.

Discovering the Monster Within

We weren't the only ones who had problems with our children in the eighties. My sister Bev's were far worse. Her's were a source of pain for the entire family.

After her father's suicide, Bev's daughter, Lori, was a handful. In and out of trouble, she tried to run away from home, ran with a fast crowd and was into alcohol and drugs at an early age. Lori, who was four months pregnant, and her husband Ron lived with Bev from the time they were married until the baby, Kristina, was born. Ron left shortly after that, and Beverly took over the job of trying to raise the child. Two years later, Lori died in a horrible automobile accident. Smelling the blood of a lawsuit like a shark, Ron reappeared. At the courts request, Ron married the woman he was living with and got custody of Kristina.

Beverly was desperate to get the child back and spent a great deal of money she didn't really have on lawyer's fees. I listened and tried to be supportive. I wanted desperately to help her financially but wasn't in a position to do so. The guilt nearly drove me out of my mind.

Ron took off again, and Kristina's stepmother rejected her. At age twelve, a good family legally adopted her. They gave her the support, discipline and instruction she needed as well as a secure environment. When she turned eighteen, she took the new car her adopted parents gave her, all the cash from the lawsuit and disappeared. She is living nearby, but we don't know where. We love her and still feel the loss.

The whole episode reaffirmed my, me-at-the-center-of-the-world, philosophy. Could I have done more? Perhaps we should have adopted her. We really couldn't afford another child, but we would have managed. Would it have mattered, or was she tainted with so many Archer dysfunctional genes nothing could have helped her. I don't know. All I remember is the anger. I was angry at myself for being so helpless. I was angry with Lori for dying and Kristina for leaving. I was angry with the pain my sister was feeling. Now, my only wish is that Kristina is safe and happy.

Death continued to stalk us and the next year, Dad Burkley began to lose his courageous battle with cancer. We made countless trips to see him, and watching this brave man waste away broke my heart. Our last visit was four days before he died, and he had to be kept upright in a chair. He was so full of fluid that if he laid down there was a danger of him drowning in his own secretions. Why couldn't I help him? What kind of nurse was I? Despite the fact that his fate was in God's hands, not mine, I could still find a way to feel guilty about it.

The day he died, we pulled Calvin from school and headed for Cleveland. When we arrived, Art's mother had already had his father cremated! Art and I were crushed. We never had a chance to say goodbye, and we never got over it.

Carolyn graduated from college and pursued her calling to go to Europe. She departed for Poland, Czechoslovakia and Romania. It was difficult for me, and I constantly worried about her. To help keep me occupied, Carolyn gave me a job before she left.

There are no salaries when you work for the Campus Crusade for Christ. And, you have no time to work an outside job. You are expected to garner support from parents, family and friends. They give you money, and in return, you report back to them on your work via a newsletter. A continued plea for more money is the centerpiece of each epistle. Carolyn supplied the content, but I became editor, publisher and distributor of her letters. I typed them up on Art's computer. That generated frequent calls to him when I ran into problems with the infernal machine. He was always patient with me, but the incidents fueled the flames of my inadequacy.

It was something I could do for her, and was glad to do it. I addressed envelopes, licked stamps and was happy to do it. Well, I didn't really lick stamps. I used a damp cloth to moisten both the stamps and the envelope flaps. No telling how many calories might be in all that glue. Unfortunately, most of the time, the contributions didn't cover all the costs, and the parents of the workers end up footing the bill. It was no different in our case.

Overwhelmed by all that had happened, Art suffered his first panic attack that year. Short of breath, he was rushed to the hospital and sequestered in the cardiac unit to rule out a heart attack. His heart proved healthy, but the depth of his anxiety surfaced. A psychiatrist was prescribed.

Art confided to the counselor that his major concern was my deteriorating health and weight loss. She asked Art to bring me to the next visit. As usual, I dressed in baggy clothes, including a sweat shirt, in an attempt to hide my true weight. After a few minutes of talking, the psychiatrist told Art to get off my back, I was fine. It pleased me that I exhibited the courage to stand up to him in front of someone else, but he never went back to her.

In November, Art's mom came down to guard Calvin while Art and I vacationed in Hawaii to celebrate our twenty-fifth wedding anniversary. Calvin even called on the eighteenth to wish us happy anniversary. It was great to get away. Art liked Hawaii, and seemed to relax there. Purging was more difficult, so I relied mostly on restricting intake. Too soon, it was back to reality.

After we returned, Art found a new therapist who began to juggle a series of medications. When Art described his concerns for my condition to him, he simply said, at my age, there was nothing that could be done. It would most likely be a fatal disease. Art loved me and was crying for help for both of us, and he didn't get it. Without getting help for me, Art's major problem would never be solved.

It wouldn't have mattered if the therapists had suggested treatment for me. I liked my illness. I was safe in my little box. Worthless as I was, I deserved no better. So, I ate and purged.

On his seventeenth birthday, Cal was walking to school, on a snowy day, with a young woman. He had to cross a set of railroad tracks near a milk plant where freeway exit and entrance ramps entered a busy highway. Snow was heaped at the edge of the tracks, and a driver, who had only cleared a small patch on his icy window, turned onto the freeway ramp and didn't see Cal. When he saw the car coming, Calvin pushed the young woman out of the way. She fell down, but was uninjured. The car struck, Calvin.

Descent into Purgatory

Racing to the hospital, I had no idea how badly he was hurt. As is my nature, I thought the worst and prayed that he wouldn't die, as guilt riddled me as bullets might have. Why didn't I drive him to school when the weather was this bad? The fact that he would never have allowed it couldn't diminish my need to feel guilty about it.

Art and I arrived at the hospital filled with horror and anger that our child had been struck by a car. Even before we saw Cal, the police told us that the accident should not have happened and suggested we had good grounds for a lawsuit. As it turned out, aside from assorted cuts and bruises, Cal had damage to his knee that required arthroscopic surgery. In time, he fully recovered. He was lucky, and we were thankful the injury was not more serious.

Encouraged by people we talked too, we followed the police officer's advice and filed a lawsuit against the driver of the car. We won the suit, and put the money away for Calvin's college education. But, the trauma of the process of the suit stretched my inadequate reserves of energy to the limit. If I had it to do over again, I probably wouldn't file a suit. I don't think the reward was worth the toll it took on me. That's right! I feel guilty about the suit.

That year, David moved back home to participate in The University of Akron's engineering co-op program. He worked for a company in nearby Canton while attending classes at the university. It was difficult for us, because David had gotten used to independent living.

We solved many of the problems by making him get his own phone line and insisting that he inform us when he would be home for meals. The problem for me was the insecurity it fostered. I was never sure when he was going to pop in, and I couldn't get caught purging.

Art had a more difficult time with it. If David was home, Art tended to treat him like he did when David was in high school. He always wanted to know where David was and what he was doing. This caused significant friction in the house, and I had to be careful not to choose sides. Personalizing their problem, I fretted because I couldn't make the situation better. The climate was explosive, and it took a further toll on my strained psyche.

Once, Art got so mad at David that he decided to throw him out of the house. In a huff, he started to move David's belongings from his basement room, starting with David's exercise weights. After three trips up and down the stairs with three hundred pounds of weights tossed into the back yard, I pleaded with David to apologize for what he had done so his father wouldn't die of a heart attack. I don't think Art really wanted him to leave, but he made his point. We can laugh about the incident, now.

Unfortunately, Art's added stress spilled over into our relationship. His depression slowly worsened, and his temper shortened. The watch-throwing personality I observed the second time I met his father returned with a vengeance. I felt like I was living with Attila the Hun.

Was I? No, I wasn't. Because of my inferiority, I had been deferring to Art for all decisions. With time, the safety of that arrangement became confining, but I still needed the victimization it produced. The internal conflict planted a seed of anger that I lacked the skills to put into the proper perspective. I began to think that Art made all the decisions because he thought I was a complete dolt. That caused the anger to boil, and I became a hostile victim. For the next few years I put the love of my life through hell. It only added to his problem. Why couldn't I see what I was doing to him? One of the tentacles of the ED personality was over my eyes, and it blinded me.

With nowhere else to turn, we went to a marriage counselor. Art's anger was a cry for help. In a one-on-one session with the counselor, Art broached my eating disorder. Although I couldn't see it, my physical appearance was reflecting the extent of the abuse I had heaped upon myself. I was approaching the skin and bones stage of the disease. Art was told by the counselor to leave me alone, I was fine.

During the late summer, my mother was suffering from pain and numbness in one of her legs, and it was getting worse. She always wanted me to take her for the tests because of my medical knowledge. At least

I was good for small things in her life. Summer dragged into fall, and after dozens of trips and tests we were no closer to an answer.

Ray's seventieth birthday came, and Mom wasn't able to do much for him because of the pain in her legs. She did get him a birthday card. As was his custom, when he had trouble sleeping, he sat dozing in his recliner in the living room. Making coffee, she brought it into the room along with the card and began to sing 'Happy Birthday' to him. Ray never saw the card. He had died peacefully in the chair an hour earlier.

His unexpected death devastated the family. Ray had been so good to Mom, and now he was gone, and she was alone and frightened. What was I going to do? How would I take care of her? I was never a good daughter, and I'd be an even worse one now. I was so upset, I couldn't eat a thing, much to ED's satisfaction.

Ray's funeral was October twentieth, and sometime between there and Halloween, my phone rang at five in the morning. My hysterical mother sobbed with pain on the other end of the line and begged me to help her. I was concerned and elated. Her pain caused the nurse in me to be concerned, and the daughter was elated that her mother had finally reached out to her. Leaping out of bed, I dressed and ran to the car.

By the time I reached Interstate Route 90, the snow began. A storm born over the shallow waters of Lake Erie bore down on its eastern shore as an impenetrable, icy curtain. Within fifteen minutes, I was in a complete white-out. No sky, no road, no cars were visible. Though I knew this road like the back of my hand, I was lost in a swirling world of white.

Terrified, I cried aloud, "God, I can't do this by myself. Help me find Mom's house!"

Creeping slowly forward, I was afraid to stop. I might freeze to death, and there would be nobody to help Mom. I wasn't worried about myself, only her. Praying constantly, I pressed forward.

An eternity later, God sent a mighty gust of wind, as He had done when the Hebrew's crossed the Red Sea. For an instant, visibility was normal before the white shawl wrapped itself around me again, blotting out everything. In that instant, I spied the exit I needed.

By the time I reached Mom's house, everyone was frantic. The storm's fury was described in vivid detail by bored weather forecasters who finally had something exciting to broadcast. Mom had tears of relief mixed with her tears of pain, and Art was ecstatic when he heard my voice on the phone. I managed to get an ambulance for Mom and took her to the hospital. The next day, they did emergency surgery on her herniated disc.

Reflecting on that harrowing journey, my relief and gratitude to my Heavenly Father was genuine. To this point in my life I had been a lip-service Christian who said the words but denied the power. I knew there was a God, but denied the love that He would give to even me if I would just accept it. This was the first inkling for me that maybe God did have the power to change lives. Could he change mine? Did he really care about *me*? Was Carolyn right? I wouldn't allow myself to accept that, yet. I was not worthy of such love. Didn't you have to do things to earn love? I never realized that God's love was a free gift, and that He loves me just as I am.

The urgent care center closed, too, and I was out of a job. Fortunately, I landed a job with a new medical delivery system in our community and was sent to Columbus, Ohio for training. I would be in charge of training people in centers all over our county.

Plunging into the job I gave it my usual one hundred ten percent. Realizing I would need nourishment to drive, I took salads to work. It was exhausting, and the pay was poor. After a year, I asked for a raise, and they denied it. Since I was making less than I would have working at a hospital, I quit and migrated to a psychiatric hospital to work, not to be admitted.

After his back injury, and upon entering high school, Cal became less of a problem. Cal became an accomplished trumpeter, and we bribed him into joining the marching and concert bands, and a talented jazz band group at school called the Gold Tones. Music allowed him to enjoy school, but he still hated to practice. He also was desperate to drive, and we bribed him with driver's education to get a B average. It worked.

Mom had her first heart attack in February of that year. It was a serious one, and it was touch and go for a bit. Finally, the doctor told us she would live and asked us if we could be with her every day, or every other day for encouragement.

In my everlasting quest to be the perfect daughter, I accepted the doctor's request as my holy grail. I continued to take care of my family, work full time and to travel to Painesville frequently to either transport my sisters to Mom's or stay with Mom myself. Dave was busy doing his own thing and had no interest in helping with her. His flock at his church needed him more.

Later that year, Mom had her second coronary. Again, she survived, but now needed full time care. Beverly moved in with her, and it was Godsend to all of us. I could stop my frantic trips to Mom's. Linda could have her life back, and Beverly, who was about to be evicted from her home, would have a place to live.

My manic behavior fueled Art's depression, and a new therapist came on the scene with the same old advice for him. In answer to Art's question about the major problem in his life, the therapist responded, "There's no need to waste time on her. There is no cure for her disease, and she is beyond hope. You just need to worry about yourself."

He completed his sage advice by treating Art with a series of medications that nearly destroyed him and us. The major source of Art's depression was me. I was killing myself and was unwilling or unable to stop it. I'm not sure if the therapists didn't know what to do with me and avoided the issue, or they failed to realize the genesis of Art's illness. Either way, it was tragic.

By now, I was over the edge. I had reached the point where I was *terrified* of food. Food was the enemy. If I took one bite of food, I might want another. Salads, raw vegetables and dry cereals were the only safe things. The sight of any food with oil, butter or sauce not only revolted me, but made me afraid. It was dangerous to me. If I ate one bite, I would lose control of the only thing in my life I could completely control.

I also lost control of my deadliest member, my tongue. I became a sharp-tongued shrew, who had no concept of the terrible, hurtful things I said to others. Mostly, it was the cruel blows I delivered to Art. In front of our friends, I would shred Art with a venomous sentence, then smile and say, "But, I love him anyway." I learned that from my family. "She should have been a boy, but we love her anyway." Cut 'em up, but sugar coat it. That was my motto.

How much I wish I could take back the words, but I can't. I only thank God that Art, and those who truly love me, have forgiven me for them.

The other technique I honed razor sharp was denial. I denied the fact that I was slowly committing suicide. When my friend, Jack, took me aside and tried to tell me that I needed help with my problem, he said, "Pat, you know you're getting worse, and I'm concerned for you."

"I know," I replied glibly. "But, I don't need any help yet. Maybe I would someday, but not now."

I denied the way I looked. Each time I looked into a mirror, I failed to see the bag of bones I had become. Instead, I saw a plump phantom that was the figment of my distorted brain. I denied the friction in my family and that Art's depression had nothing to do with my ED.

I could deny I was destroying my marriage. I could deny anything I wanted to deny.

On the twenty-ninth of December, as I was getting ready for work, Calvin and I got into an argument. His verbal abuse of me reached its zenith that night. When he called me a fucking bitch, I lashed out at him meaning to slap him in the face.

With the reflexes of youth, Cal raised his hands in self defense, and my blow of righteous wrath struck his forearm instead. He was uninjured, but I severely sprained my thumb which required a trip to the emergency room.

Descent into Purgatory

Always the martyr, and despite the throb in my thumb, I went to work with it splinted. The shift seemed to last forever. When it was over, I went out to my car, slipped on the ice and broke my elbow! A second trip to the emergency room in twelve hours left me with another splint and a sling.

Jack and Pat Summers had invited our bridge bunch to an elegant New Year's Eve celebration. The country club was festive and the music wonderful. If I had not been trying to starve myself to death, the food would have been delectable as well. My thumb throbbed. My elbow felt as if an ice pick was imbedded in it, and I was in no mood to celebrate anything.

Most of all, I was angry. Angry with Calvin; angry with Art; angry with my life! My body and my brain were so starved for nutrition that I couldn't think straight.

As the band played, 'Auld Lang Syne,' and colorful balloons cascaded from the ceiling, I was surrounded by people who loved me, and would have done anything they could for me. Instead, I refused to admit I needed help and seethed, denied, suppressed and starved. Happy New Year!

CHAPTER 10

Descent into Hell

Accarding to Dante, after purgatory comes hell, and I gradually descended into it.

By now, I was constantly hungry, and the feeling terrified me. Before, the hunger was intermittent, but I had starved my body to the point that hunger was a living, breathing thing that tormented me day and night. I felt as if I was in the eye of a hurricane, and everything around me was spinning wildly out of control. Food consumption was all that was left. It was the delicate spider's thread that connected me to the real world. If that thread broke, I would fly into the chaos around me. My mind and body shrieked for nourishment. I was starving, and I knew it, but I was powerless to change. I would rather *die* than *gain an ounce.*

I enjoyed the role of victim. Everyone else's problems were my fault. Each of life's little tragedies was somehow the result of something I did or didn't do. My cup of guilt was always half full. One day, as I mused over a problem, I experienced an epiphany that would eventually save my life. I came to the understanding that everything that happened wasn't *always* my fault. Sometimes, my problems were caused by what others did. Armed with this "divine inspiration," I unleashed a side of my personality I never knew I possessed. I began to turn anger and guilt into hostility and venom, which I dispensed with a smile.

In keeping with my personality, I carried these traits to the extreme, and that was bad. On the good side, it was the first time in my life that I ever admitted to myself that I was a person who was worth something. I didn't always have to be at the mercy of others. Lacking acceptable skills to implement these new feelings, I leaked them out like acid from a cracked battery.

The fractured elbow ruined more than New Year's Eve. Since it was my dominant arm, I found it difficult to purge. Swooning back into the arms of my old lover, restriction, I added a new and dangerous twist, laxatives. When Art retired, he would be under foot more and purging presented a logistical problem. Laxatives were the answer.

Fatigue was now my constant companion, but I continued to deny both the hunger and the fatigue. I had burned the candle at both ends for years, and now one wick had been extinguished and the other was sputtering. I liked to brag about how little sleep I got, and how much I was able to do as a result. Now, with all my energy reserves gone, I felt as if I were a hundred years old.

Art and I traveled back to Hawaii because we had fallen in love with the place, and prayed that a little time in Paradise might solve some of our problems. It didn't. I found simple walking to be exhausting. One day, after only three blocks, I felt as if I had just finished the Bataan Death March. We stopped at a McDonalds so I could rest, and I ordered a glass of milk. It was sour! I nearly cried as the symbolism of it struck me. I was worn out. ED had won not only the battle but the war as well. My whole existence was as sour as the milk in my cup. I was in big trouble with no idea how to get out of it.

Zero birthdays tend to be tougher than ones that end with numbers. To be forty-nine is not so bad. Then, the zero birthday sneaks up and everything changes. To ease the pain of my fifth zero birthday, Art took me to Columbus, Ohio for the weekend. As we sat in an elegant restaurant, I felt bold enough to pose a question that had been eating at me for months.

"Art," I began hesitantly, "what's going on?"

When he replied with a quizzical look, I pressed on. "You haven't touched me for over a year. Our physical relationship is non-existent. Is there someone else?" I asked my heart racing as I feared his answer.

"No, there has never been another woman," he replied, his voice quivering with the sting of the unfounded accusation.

"Is it me? Is it the way I look? Am I repulsive to you?"

"Yes, you are," he said bitterly.

Art was hurt that I would accuse him of infidelity; terrified that I was going to die; angry with me for not realizing my situation; angry with himself for not being able to help me. He hoped his scathing response might shock me into doing something about my fatal condition.

Unfortunately, it didn't work. When I looked into the mirror, I still saw a chunky creature that desperately needed to lose weight. I was too fat. That was it! If I could lose a little more, he wouldn't find me repulsive. I couldn't see the true reflection of a malnourished scarecrow that rivaled the best skeleton in a Halloween parade. I was hurt by his comment, but wasn't bitter about it. I believe a part of my subconscious mind agreed with his assessment.

Besides my problems, Art suffered from physical ailments that wore on him as well. After months of battling a sour stomach and heart burn that was unrelieved by antacids and attributed to nervous tension, he was hospitalized. They found a bleeding ulcer near the junction of the esophagus and the stomach. Fortunately, the biopsy was negative for cancer. With appropriate prescription therapy, he felt considerable relief, although the symptoms did not completely abate.

A year later, Art's symptoms returned with a vengeance, and he had to be re-hospitalized for another complete evaluation including more biopsies. My niece Liz's wedding took placed on June 29th while Art was in the hospital. He encouraged me to go without him.

Descent into Hell

I took my mother-in-law to the wedding. After the ceremony, I slammed the car door on my leg and sliced it open. I drove myself to the emergency room where stitches were required to close it. By the time I arrived at the reception, dinner was over. Hooray! I wouldn't have to invent reasons not to eat. Over a couple of glasses of champagne, I visited with everyone at the party. Busy little social butterfly! Busy little girl! Life was good, at least for ED.

As the Fourth of July approached, instead of the usual fireworks, a bomb was dropped on the Burkley family. Art's latest biopsy was positive for cancer. He would need surgery, and it was scheduled for the eighth.

I spent the days with Art and continued working my full shift at night. Despite the constant fatigue, I pushed myself even harder, and on the two days before the surgery, I didn't sleep at all. I ate barely enough to sustain me. Why I didn't die, I will never know!

Art's tumor was confined to the esophagus, and Dr. Mike Flynn was able to remove the tumor, part of the esophagus and part of the stomach, leaving no tumor behind. He was able to reconnect the good esophagus with disease free stomach, so Art would eventually be able to eat normally. Then, he began the long, slow road to recovery.

On the eighth postoperative day, my friend Mary Jane, from the osteopathic hospital, who was now living in Arizona, came to visit. I met her for lunch and was shocked when I saw her. Although she still weighed two hundred pounds, she had lost over a hundred. Mary Jane had cancer of the pancreas and had come to say goodbye. She had undergone all the chemo she could stand.

"I'm not spending the rest of my life over a toilet bowl," she said, in typical Mary Jane fashion.

Despite the gravity of her situation, and the things that she said to me, I didn't grasp what she was saying. I was so wrapped up in Art's problem, and in myself, that I didn't understand that she was telling me she was going to die.

Discovering the Monster Within

During Art's long and difficult recovery, I felt a great deal of pressure. I was filled with free-floating anxiety and anger. I couldn't put my finger on the exact cause of the feeling, so I tried to escape from it. I found a new source of comfort that coincidently supplied a little nutrition. It was V-Eight vegetable juice and vodka! It never occurred to me that I might follow my father's predilection for addiction to the alcohol. After all, it was just a temporary escape from the pressure. Besides, it had calories in it, and I wasn't so tired all the time.

Art faced his uncertain future with dread. In his usual fashion, he turned his anxiety into anger, something he could handle better. Meanwhile I was a first-rate, sharp-tongued shrew, and he couldn't make me see that I was starving to death.

In an attempt to break our vicious spiral, he took me on a short cruise to the Bahamas. Art had no energy at all, and spent most of the time ensconced in a deck chair. I did my own thing, avoided the wonderful food they offered four times a day, and had a grand time. When we returned home, I found out that while I was having a great time, Mary Jane died and was buried. The reality of what she tried to tell me hit home. ED was gleeful over the amount of grief I heaped upon myself. A month after our return, Art retired, but continued to work under contract until August of the next year.

Carolyn was getting ready to leave on her European mission trip when Calvin, and his girlfriend, Tina, who had been living together, decided to get married. They had become deeply involved in their church, and their current living arrangement bothered them. They wanted Carolyn to be in the wedding, so they hastily put together plans for a simple ceremony. On July tenth, nineteen ninety-three, they were married. I couldn't have been happier. Calvin had outgrown his teen-aged rebellion, and had become a fine, responsible young man. And, Art and I both dearly loved Tina.

The newlyweds returned to their home, Carolyn left for Slovakia, and David, after flitting back and forth between California and Arizona, settled in Arizona. Our nest was truly empty for the first time. So, we decided to take a cruise with Linda and Dan to the Caribbean.

Forced into the formality of mealtime aboard cruise ships, I ate only the appetizer and the salad. Since we ate with the same people every day, the other couples noticed how little I ate. When we parted at the end of the cruise, my tablemates told me they would pray for me. I was never sure if they thought I had a terminal disease, or just realized that I was starving myself. Either way, I rationalized away their concern and continued down my merry road toward disaster.

To add to his woes, Art became his mother's guardian. To facilitate her care, we moved her to an Akron facility closer to us. When moving day arrived, Art refused to take the day off from his consulting job, so I had to move her myself. This once domineering woman was like a lost child. She had to drag her ironing board, cooking utensils and cleaning equipment with her, even though she would never use them. Every five minutes as we drove down the highway she asked, "Are we there yet?"

Mom Burkley was angry, too. She was angry with Art; angry with me; angry with the world. By the time I had her settled in, I was furious with Art. How could he have stuck me with this unpleasant task? Instead of expressing my feelings to him, I internalized the anger and fueled ED's next bonfire.

Our new level of responsibility for Mom Burkley placed even more strain on an already strained relationship. She was beginning to lose her mental faculties, and Art found that troubling. So, he turned most of the visitation duties over to me. I tried to be upbeat about it, but it was difficult.

Occasionally, I tried to take her out of the facility for lunch, just to give her a break. Her behavior made them an ordeal. She had a number of nasty tricks that included throwing biscuits across the restaurant. When we were walking out after lunch, she had a habit of picking up the tip money left for the waitresses. That one really embarrassed me. I kept up the lunches as long as I could stand them, but the resentment was enormous. Steaming, I internalized my anger and allowed it to eat at me.

Of all the things ED did to me, the worst was the effect it had on Art. He feared for my life and was powerless to help me. The fear-fed anger it produced left him in a state of constant, smoldering depression that was incapacitating. My normally active, energetic mate was capable of doing nothing constructive. He had a constant fine tremor from medication that was so bad he couldn't even read. We consulted a new psychiatrist.

The face was new, but the result was the same. When Art broached the real cause of his mental depression, she told him that I was just fine, to leave me alone and work on his own problems. She didn't understand that I *was* his major problem.

She placed him on a series of mood elevators and antidepressants. They did very little for him, except produce side effects. Art had friends, but wouldn't reach out to them, or burden them with his problems. Our really good friends stood helplessly by, unable to intervene, and not knowing how to help us. This was one of the bleakest periods in our lives.

My condition was underscored by our next visit to Hawaii. We went to the big island of Hawaii with Linda and Dan. At the National Park, the rangers conduct a forty-five minute informational walk around the caldera of Kilauea. I started the walk, passed out and fell flat on my face. I was too exhausted to continue the hike.

They revived me, and I tried to leave. When I got up, I fell again. I was too weak to stand. Art asked me if I was drunk. That really hurt me, because it was certainly a legitimate question. My alcohol consumption had increased significantly. In truth, the majority of my calories probably came from alcohol.

The second fall ripped open my leg, and when we had deposited Linda and Dan at the hotel, Art took me to the emergency room. Thirteen stitches closed the paper-thin skin over my leg. With no fat at all to send healing blood vessels to the area, it didn't heal very well.

Descent into Hell

Despite this disastrous day, I insisted that we continue with the trip. I was fine. There was nothing to worry about. It's unimaginable to me now that I could have felt that way. I was dying by inches, my marriage was in shambles, and all I could do was smile, and starve and deny that any of it was happening.

Others died around me during this time. Besides my friend, Mary Jane, Sue, my old pal from nursing school, found her husband, "Coupe," was critically ill. My nephew Todd lost his first wife. After she died, Todd tried to get custody of the children who had been living with her. He asked Linda and me to be character witnesses. We went to the courthouse in Ashtabula County, but the hearing was delayed. I called home to tell Art we were running late, and he told me his mother had passed away. Her death added to Art's depression. With all that death around me, it should have made me consider my own mortality, but it didn't.

Since I had restricted my intake of food as much as an anorexic can, purged in the best tradition of the bulimic, and added laxatives to the mix like a suicidal fool, I found that alcohol provided a little relief, so I continued to drink.

With no where else to go, I turned toward God for an answer. I went to church and Bible study regularly. I sought to find a way to change. Although the answer was right there in front of me, I couldn't see it. I also started seeing a counselor at the Chapel on Fir Hill where we went to church. It was a waste of time, because I wasn't ready to be helped.

Art continued to suffer from pain in his abdomen. Our fear was that the cancer had returned. It reached the point that exploratory surgery was undertaken. They removed fourteen inches of both large and small bowel where inflammatory diverticulitis had plastered them together. Thank God all was benign.

The day he went into surgery, Art was nearly impossible to live with. He was afraid that recovery from this surgery would be as bad as the recovery from his esophageal surgery. Three days post-op, minus the grinding pain in his guts that had been slowly consuming him, he was a different person. Neither of us had realized how much the relentless pain had affected him. This time, his recovery was more normal.

I knew that Sue's husband was ill, so I called her to see how he was doing, and to share my good news. She told me that his funeral was the next day, and asked if I would be able to attend. I felt an odd mixture of sadness and relief. Her loss made me sad, but at the same time I was relieved that I still had Art. In keeping with tradition, I felt guilty that Art was alive, and her husband was dead.

It was impossible to believe that our lives could have been any bleaker. Art was struggling through another major surgery while battling his anxieties and depressions. I was starving in mind and body and drinking way too much. Our marriage was on the rocks, and I was scared to death that Art might die, or he might be driven away by our continuing problems. Just when I had convinced myself that things couldn't be any worse, a tragedy slashed into our lives and threatened to chop us both to ribbons.

June seventh, nineteen ninety-seven, is a date I will never forget. It lives in shock and horror for me as clearly as the World Trade Center Attack does for the nation. I remember the date for two reasons. First, David had decided that although he had a successful career in engineering, he might want to go to medical school. The Medical College Admission Test was required, and was to be administered that day, in Cleveland. The second reason I remember the date is because it was the day I lost my daughter!

David had come to Ohio to take his test, and Cal and Tina had come over to the house. I was busy making their favorite cookies for my two sons when the phone rang. When I heard Carolyn's voice, I was excited. She was back from Europe, and we hadn't seen her since Christmas of nineteen ninety-six. I told her what was going on and added that it was a perfect day, and she was the only thing missing.

My smile turned to a grimace of pain as she told me that she had been seeing a Christian counselor, and that she had some issues with me. As long as these issues were unresolved, she would not be communicating with me. She said I was controlling, and she felt unsafe around me. When she came home, she felt unsafe, so she would not be coming home again.

As I grope for a word to describe my feelings, none comes to mind even now. Nothing I can think of is terrible enough. The only words I could stammer were, "How can I help?"

To my shock, she had the gall to answer that I could send her money. The sessions with the counselor were expensive, and the costs were straining her budget. In the same breath, she set down rules for any further contact.

First, these rules were only for me. Art was free to contact her as he pleased. It made my heart feel as if an ice pick had been shoved into it. I expected to find blood on my shirt when I looked down. I could write to her, but not phone her or try to talk to her. Without further explanation, she hung up on me.

I sat there staring at the phone as if it were a snake that had just bitten me. My whole world crashed down around me. She will never understand the kind of pain she inflicted on me that day. When I told Art about it, he was as shocked, hurt and bewildered by it all as I was.

She had stated that Art could contact her, so he called her. In fact he called several times over the next weeks. Despite her benevolent promise to communicate with him, she never answered the phone or returned any of the messages he left for her.

Next, we both wrote to her, and she did answer some of the correspondence. Since we never talked to her personally, we pieced together the following scenario. For reasons that remain unclear to us, she felt the need to seek a counselor. She chose a Christian counselor, whose name or credentials was never supplied to us. Through a series of sessions that involved regressive therapy, taking her back to her childhood and unlocking so-called repressed memory, she was convinced that some of the most ludicrous things imaginable had happened to her.

Her letters were skillfully crafted. She felt I was controlling, but she brought the process to a new level. While attempting to validate her position, she skillfully tried to make any lack of communication our fault. She set down ridiculous rules that we were to follow if we contacted her. Then, she told us it was our choice. If we didn't follow her impossible rules, then we were choosing not to communicate with her, and it would be our fault.

When she did get around to telling us what she had been "helped to remember," had she not so truly believed them, they would have been darkly humorous. She claimed that since the age of four or five, Art's father had been systematically raping her, and that it lasted for several years. Carolyn goes on to accuse a pastor of running a cult at a church. She was taken there, and the men and women passed her around in "bazaar, sadistic, sexual rituals." In her recollections, she clearly sees the faces of the men who abused her. "This is as clear to me as the pen I'm writing with now," she states in her letter describing the events. Though not directly, she insinuates that we permitted these atrocities to transpire.

These accusations are so dreadfully false that I feel embarrassed to deny them, but I must. As God is our witness, we know that these accusations are figments of a lie in the fragile psyche of a troubled girl. None of them ever happened.

For starters, when she was a child, Carolyn was seldom alone with Art's father long enough for any of these atrocities to have taken place. Art's mom and dad always did everything together, and she almost never left Dad Burkley alone with her long enough for the activities Carolyn thinks she remembers. David and Calvin were usually there with her, and their memories are of TV, munchies and loving, doting grandparents.

My daughter has remembered a number of things that never happened, and forgotten a number of things that did happen. Carolyn is music major and I don't think she ever took any anatomy classes. It is not surprising that she doesn't know the near impossibility of an adult male raping a four or five year old girl without inflicting physical damage to vagina or rectum that would require the care of a skilled surgeon to repair. Particularly if she was raped by multiple adult males as she thinks she remembers.

The major point she has forgotten was the state of Dad Burkley's health. When she accuses him of these deviant sexual activities, he had the prostate cancer that would eventually kill him. The radiation therapy to the prostate, and the hormonal manipulation that went on for a dozen years, rendered him physically unable to perform the criminal acts she so clearly recalls.

Another thing she neglected to remember was the absence of physical manifestations of abuse. She had no bruises, lacerations, tears, or other signs of injury visible on her body. If she was indeed involved in "sadistic sexual rituals," there would have been visible signs of it. There were not. At the age she claimed this happened, they would have been so evident they could not have been ignored.

Unfortunately, she has also forgotten our friends and neighbors. They were intelligent, and included elementary teachers who could spot abuse a mile away in the children they taught. And, not just the physical signs, but the emotional ones, too. One was a physician who knew the physical and emotional aspects of abused children. None of them saw anything to suggest Carolyn was being abused. When we told our friends about her accusations, they were as flabbergasted as we were.

She also has forgotten her playmates. Summer attire in Ohio included shorts, t-shirts and tank-tops that would have advertised bruises and lacerations as a billboard advertises pizza. No one ever saw any.

Aside from the pain she caused us, she damaged Art in a particular hurtful way. He loves children, and is one of the kindest, most patient teachers I have ever seen. A master woodworker, he is also an artist in stained glass. He loves to share his talents with others, particularly children. Although his only crime is loving his daughter, she has made him leery of contact with other children. If his own daughter could make such a preposterous charge, what damage could another child do? How sad. Fortunately, he has two wonderful daughters-in-law who know the truth about the man and are helping to heal the residual scars left by her unfounded attack.

Interestingly, despite the fact that she accused Art's father of the atrocities, she proposed to remain in touch with Art while treating me as the leper. I could not fathom that. I have three children that I love more than my own life, and one of them tells me she is afraid of me. It makes my heart ache when I think about it. Despite her warning, I wrote to her and begged her for specifics about what I had done. I told her that whether she liked it or not, I was her mother, and I felt she owed me an explanation.

In her reply, she began by telling me that she owed me nothing. She had never asked to be born. Her birth was my choice, not hers, and she owed me nothing. I wonder what runs through her mind when she reads the commandment to honor her father and mother.

She went on to attribute to me a Jekyll and Hyde personality that is no closer to reality than her satanic rituals. Charging I called her a "selfish fucking bitch," she claims that in a hysterical fit of anger, I then threw a plate of food against the wall.

Did I tell her she was selfish? I probably did, because she was. Did I embellish it with profanity? That's unlikely, because that's not me. The only time I clearly remember those words were on New Year's Eve when I was the recipient of the epithet, not the originator of it. Art and the boys remember things that way, too.

I'm afraid the food-throwing episode is true. Embarrassed, I had to clean up the mess myself. But, I never touched her at that time. Art, who misses nothing, knew it happened. I never tried to hide anything from him.

Recalling lying on the floor in a ball to escape blows from a wooden spoon, she claims to have been the target of repeated beatings by her half-crazed maniac mother. I admit to being a parent of the seventies. I never discussed philosophies of behavior with a two year old, and I spanked my children when they were naughty. The key word is spanked. I never beat anyone.

Descent into Hell

A wooden spoon might make a nice paddle, but I *never* used it for that. I never left a bruise or permanent red mark on any of my children. My only weapon was my hand, and the only target was a bottom. She knows that, and so does everyone who knew our children and us during the time in question. Again she has forgotten that such beatings would leave unmistakable marks on her for teachers, neighbors and the other children to see. She had none.

One thing was certain. I punished the children equally. Perhaps it bothered her more than it did her brothers. Cal and David don't remember ever being *beaten* with anything, let alone a wooded spoon. She remembers it differently than the way it happened. Apparently, she remembers a lot of her childhood differently than it actually happened. I believe that's the case here, too.

She also remarked that I only expressed my rage with the children, turning it off the moment Art came in the door. I'm afraid she gives me credit for acting ability I never possessed. I usually internalized my anger, and that never changed. On rare occasion when I did lose it, I was back in control almost immediately. Where Art was concerned, my heart was always on my sleeve, and he knew me to well to be fooled if I had tried to deceive him as she charged.

I'm afraid what she did see was my Ms. Fixit personality. I tried to please Art in everything and it showed. Since I had no emotions of my own, I had to make Art happy so I could be happy. I had to make things perfect for him so they would be perfect for me. There's no way she could have understood that. For that, I am sorry.

My heart was particularly heavy when she told me that she had lain awake nights worrying about whether or not I might die. She knew I was starving myself to death, and she was afraid I might succeed. On this charge, Carolyn, I am guilty. My problem with ED has caused enormous pain to all those who love me. For that, I am eternally sorry. I knew she was right, but at the time she said it to me, I still couldn't force myself to seek help. That's how far gone I was.

Discovering the Monster Within

Carolyn responded to one of Art's letters with terms for future contact. He was never to question the fact that she was abused; never loose his temper or use profanity when they talked, which they haven't since before that fateful phone call; and respect her right to say no. Art's heart was broken, but he couldn't live by rule number one. To write or talk to her under such conditions did not allow the real issue to be discussed and gave acquiescence to the lie. I feel her only reason was to feed her need for control. Art refused to play the game, and I supported his courageous decision.

I am filled with sorrow when I see the sad little girl behind the words. She is making herself comfortable at our emotional expense. I understand that, because I used ED the same way. In letters filled with accusations about how horrible we are, she asks us for money to continue the therapy that is tearing us apart as a family. When she sets down impossible rules for communication, she asks us to send her a favorite dollhouse. I believe my beloved daughter does need help. I only pray that she does not take forty years to find it, as I did.

Her actions also impacted our faith. I remember one of the last times I saw Carolyn and my brother Dave together. They literally glowed as they discussed different interpretations of Biblical passages and exchanged ideas about God. I envied that. But, they also shut out everyone and everything that did not share their charismatic view of divine love and redemption. I didn't envy that. Art and I both have trouble with a doctrine that would excommunicate family and give lip service to the all powerful love and forgiveness of God but refuse to practice it in their own lives.

During this terrible time, Art said to me, "If this is how your God is, I don't want any part of Him. It hurts too much!"

Other than a few letters within several months of the break off, mostly requesting money to support her work with the Campus Crusade, we seldom heard from Carolyn directly. Reflecting on the situation, I can understand her behavior somewhat. I believe she felt that her life was as out of control as I felt mine seemed to be. I chose an eating disorder to control mine. She chose her own way. In the end, both methods severely damaged the family who loved us both. Unfortunately, she has traded one form of control for another. She has given control to her therapist and is building her emotional life on a lie. I can only pray that she will not fall as far, or as long as I did before she discovers the truth.

She stays in touch with her brothers, and we have encouraged them to keep in touch with her. Through them, we understand she married a man who already had children, and she is doing counseling in the Christian community. We hope that she is happy, and we pray that one-day, before it is too late for us, that the same God we both serve will show her the truth, and she will be reunited with us.

How does one reconcile the living death of a child? Carolyn is alive, but she is dead to us. Since this devastation, Art and I have renewed our faith. We serve a kind, compassionate God, full of love and forgiveness that reaches out to the whole world, not just to a select few. We have forgiven her the pain she has caused us. A lie can only damage you if you let it. Whatever the outcome, His will be done.

I also believe that God controls my life, and when an adverse event occurs, there is, at the very least, a lesson to be learned. As Art and I reflected on this time, we both came to the realization that we were at the bottom of the barrel. And, for the first time, I considered the possibility that I was in desperate need of help.

There were physical consequences to Carolyn's actions as well. Physically, I was on the edge of the grave, and as I turned to contemplate crawling back out of it, she threw dirt in my face. Art was pushed to the edge of irreversible depression as he battled cancer and gut grinding diverticulitis. Our marriage had deteriorated. Working nights six days a week eased that pain, and meant we only slept in the same bed one day a week.

This also meant that Art was at home and awake during the day. Purging was out of the question, so I dusted off my anorexic behavior. Since Carolyn had turned what was left of my world upside down, I *had* to stay in control of my eating. Once again, I placed a cartridge in the cylinder and spun the revolver's chamber. Placing my ED gun against my temple in Russian-roulette fashion, I increased the laxatives in my daily menu. The hammer dropped on an empty chamber, for the moment.

After much soul searching, and Art having survived cancer for five years, we agreed that a new start was in order. Studying various retirement areas, we decided on a visit to Arizona. At least we would be closer to David there. Contacting a realtor, we boarded the plane with a modicum of hope in our hearts.

Once we met with the relater, our hopes were dashed. She was unprepared for our visit, and incapable of showing us anything at all useful. We did have a nice visit with David. Otherwise, the trip was a bust.

On the way home, I was as depressed as I can ever remember being. I had no daughter, no marriage and the holidays were coming. Fortunately, David and his fiancée Kathy planned to visit us over Christmas and New Years. Otherwise, they might have been too much to bear.

One more sorrow awaited us before we returned from Arizona. A friend of our son David had a tragic bout with cancer. Charles had been in the Gold Tones with David, and was a frequent visitor to our home. While in college, he had been diagnosed with a brain tumor. He endured exhaustive therapy, and went into remission long enough to finish college. Several years later, the cancer returned with a vengeance.

Charles' parents could not handle this tragedy, and we became Charles' surrogate parents. Art became very close to the boy, and took him to and from his therapy sessions. We knew the end was near, but did not expect him to die while we were in Arizona, but he did. It was a blow to us both, but particularly Art. His depression deepened.

The following January, Art asked me, "How about Las Vegas?"

Las Vegas? Wasn't that just one big gambling casino in the middle of nowhere? Did people really live there? Things were so bad I said, "Why not."

It had some advantages. David would be eight hours away. Housing was economical, and taxes practically non-existent, or so we thought.

Descent into Hell

The weather was hot enough that I would never be cold again. Holding our breath, we consulted another real estate agent.

This time, we got a winner. We fell in love with the area, and the house we chose proved to be perfect for us. On February twenty-third, nineteen ninety-eight, we signed the contract for the house. Filled with anticipation, we headed home to break the news to family and friends.

The news of our impending move shocked and dismayed my mother. I spent a great deal of time with her and my family while Art did nearly all the packing. It was best for both of us. Being away from each other eased the tension between us, and allowed me to control my eating. Laxative use was climbing, and I was up to several doses per day by now. I also continued to work, keeping my full time job till the very end.

In late March, David and his friend Dan came to Ohio. The movers packed the furniture, and we drove one car while David and Dan drove the other. With hope for the future, we set out for what I hoped would be a new beginning.

Once we were on the road, the togetherness of the moment dissolved into the chaos our lives had become. I now realize that most of it was my fault because of the destructive way my tortured psyche interpreted even the simplest of things.

A prime example occurred when we stopped for the night in New Mexico. In the late afternoon, Art spotted a large number of hot air balloons near our motel. "Come take a look at this," he said to me. It was a simple statement. He saw something he thought was exciting, and he wanted to share with me. Unfortunately, I interpreted it as a command. I was to come there at once and do his bidding! With reality as distorted as that, things could only get worse.

When we arrived in the Promised Land, our new home wasn't ready yet. So, we moved into a Budget Suite Hotel that would be our refuge for the next nine weeks. The close quarters became another obstacle to be overcome.

Discovering the Monster Within

Art is a detail-oriented perfectionist. He demands it of himself, as shown in the professional quality of his woodworking and stained glass. He also demands it of others who sign contracts to do work for him. Fussing over the construction of the house was right up his alley.

In the evenings, or when the weekends halted construction at the house, things got tense in our confining quarters. So, we did a lot of exploring. We simply got into the car, picked a direction and set off in search of adventure. It broke the tension and helped us familiarize ourselves with the area.

The small apartment made bulimic behavior impossible, so I restricted and upped the laxatives to shameful levels. At least I remained in control, or so I thought.

On the seventh of July, we finally took possession of our new digs. Our furniture, stored in Ohio, was delayed another three weeks, thanks to the construction delay. What furniture we did have had been purchased in Las Vegas, and we had it delivered the day we took possession. We slept on a mattress on the floor for three weeks, while David and Kathy, who came to visit and see the new house, slept on the floor.

When the furniture finally arrived, I plunged into unpacking with all the hyperactive energy I could muster. There was always one more box to unpack, one more box to take to the curb. Fatigue set in early, and on one trip to the curb with a big cardboard box, and I dropped it on my leg. The pain was intense, but like a good trooper, I bit the bullet and carried on.

My leg was nothing but malnourished skin stretched over decalcifying bone and starving muscle. The blow from the box bruised one of the muscles so severely that blood accumulated in the muscle fibers. Over the next two weeks, the bruise spread and the pain intensified. Finally, the skin ruptured releasing a cup of black blood as thick as motor-oil. It left a surface wound that wouldn't heal.

I was dispatched to the UMC burn center for treatment of my leg. I was going to church and Bible study routinely, so I used the waiting time to study the Bible. Somewhere in that Book had to be the answer to the mess my life had become.

One day, as I was leaving the UMC, the wind began to blow. Unacquainted with the fierce wind and sandstorms that plague the desert, I wandered down the street toward where the car was parked. In a matter of minutes, debris swirled around me reminiscent of Dorothy's Kansas tornado. Since I had no desire to go to Oz, I sought refuge in a nearby store.

As I struggled to traverse the few yards to safety, an orange crate propelled by the howling wind flew down the street and struck my *other leg*! Bleeding profusely, I hobbled into the store. The manager took me to the back and bandaged my dripping wound. For the next six months, I wore bandages on both legs as my famished tissue tried to repair itself.

In August, my mother died, and we went back to Ohio for the funeral. ED helped me handle the added stress in the usual fashion. Before the funeral, I asked my brother, Dave, who would be conducting the service, if I might say a few words. "No!" was his terse reply. In the end, he should have allowed me to speak.

To the dismay of everyone at the service, he said, "If I could think of anything good to say about her, I would say it. But, I can't."

Stunned, and lacking the emotional equipment to handle a confrontation with him, I didn't say anything about it for years.

Sad, depressed, discouraged, I returned to Las Vegas, and an uncertain future.

CHAPTER 11

Do or Die Time

Ifeel I was fortunate. Many anorexics do not have the support that I had during the bleakest period of my life. As Jacob wrestled with the angel in Genesis, I wrestled with my angels about control of my life and the dreadful condition that was killing me. It took two years, but the angels won.

Back in Nevada, I had time for a great deal of reflection. My brother's cruel words at Mom's funeral service still lashed at my heart like a barbed whip, and I was torn by my swirling emotions. The final years of her life had no quality. She was in diapers, with no memory, in a nursing home, and in that regard, God was merciful to take her home. It was a merciful death, and I could accept that.

What I couldn't accept was my own cowardice in the face of my brother's cruelty. Why didn't I stand up for her? Why didn't I honor her? I felt so ashamed that so many people heard only his words and not the words in my heart. I want to stand straight and tall, but more often shrink back in shame. Instead of the brilliant leaf of fall, boldly displaying its colors to the world, I'm the worthless, dry, shriveled leaf of winter, swept away by the frigid wind.

It goes back to my childhood. I learned that children, particularly females, were to be seen and not heard. Our father's daily treatment of us confirmed our status as resident non-entities. I fought the system with my mouth and my actions. The lesson was simple. If I wanted to be a person, instead of a non-entity, it would cause more pain to me and to those I loved than I felt I could endure.

Upon that sand, I built my unstable house of emotions and convinced myself that I didn't deserve to have feelings. If I expressed them, they came crashing painfully down around my ears. It was better to deny and bury them. That way, the shame was easier to bear. If I had stepped forward and demanded to pay tribute to my mother, would it have done more harm than good? I don't know, but the victim in me wouldn 't let me find out. Reverting to the survival training of my youth, I buried my brother's comments and my cowardice while ED respectfully nodded and smiled.

Unfortunately, those skills were useful while we lived in the Budget Suite. Watching my poor husband stew over the shoddy workmanship and the seemingly countless delays in the construction of our home, I was afraid that the watch throwing boy I knew so many years ago might re-appear and stay this time. His anger and sadness were more than I could bear. I was supposed to fix everything for him, and I couldn't do it. Surprise, surprise! Perhaps some time alone would be the answer.

I took lots of long, leisurely walks, and once gave Art the gift of an entire day alone. I knew that he needed it, but wasn't aware that I needed it, too. Besides, what better way to be a non-entity?

While passing a church on one of my walks, I realized that I needed an immediate church connection. In a Christian women's magazine I subscribed to, I read that Beth Moore would be holding a conference at the Canyon Ridge Church. Only three miles from where our new home was being built, the church's location was ideal. It was the perfect opportunity, and I wanted to go.

Still feeling I needed Art's permission for everything, I cleared it with him before I bought a ticket. Art drove me to the church, so I would know where it was and how to get there. It was a joyous experience, and I met many wonderful people. God directed me there. I feel certain of that.

Mother's Day Sunday was the first time I attended a service at the new church. They presented me with a beautiful red rose whose fragrance permeated the air in our tiny motel room. Tina and Cal sent me flowers, and I still have the vase they came in. Art took me to a champagne brunch to honor the day. The sky was cobalt blue, the distant mountains gleamed in the sunlight and the day was perfect. I drank the champagne but ate practically nothing at the sumptuous repast. As Auntie Maim said, "Life is a banquet, and most poor suckers out there are starving." I was a sucker that day to be sure.

There seemed an infinite supply of Christian women in the Canyon Ridge Church, and I found friends immediately. I helped start a Bible study in my home. Because of the pathologic way I interpreted and processed information, and because the resentment and anger of so many years was boiling over, I treated Art badly. I sent so many negative messages to the women in the group that I'm afraid I turned many of them against him. I made him the ogre, instead of the true monster, old ED and me. I will forever regret this, and the countless other hurts I've delivered to this good man.

The church had a special course called, "Experiencing God," and being eager for knowledge that might help me in my walk with God, I signed up. Here, was my epiphany. For the first time, I got it through my armor plated skull that *this was not about me*! Life was about God, and our relationship with Him. Ever so slowly, the focus of my life inched from inward to outward.

Most of my adult life, I have worked. At times I worked only for the money, while at other times it was for my sanity, for self-gratification, and for the love of my fellow man. I also need to work to continue to prove my father wrong. I'm not just a baby factory! I'm a good nurse! Most of the doctors I worked for told me so. I realize that God has blessed me with the talent of healing, and I must do something, even if it's only a little bit, with that marvelous gift. Bored and restless those first few weeks in Vegas, I scouted the job market, filled out a few applications and haunted the malls.

One day, I chanced into a Lemstone's Christian Book Store. While talking to the manager, I jokingly said that I would love to have a job while I was waiting for something to break in nursing. She gave me an application. I filled it out and was hired on the spot for a whopping five dollars an hour.

The wages and the crazy hours drove Art bonkers, but I have always loved working with the public and thoroughly enjoyed it. It was good for me and bad for my marriage. But, to be totally honest, I didn't see how the marriage could have gotten much worse. While working there, I met my friend Monika, one of the most important people in getting me into therapy. The job also allowed me to grow in my knowledge of God and His character, and was a booster shot for my self esteem.

Another reason for working was to earn my way. I felt the compulsion to contribute. At least if I was working, I wasn't costing Art anything. When I landed my first nursing job, it relieved the stress on the marriage considerably, and I was back doing what I felt God wanted me to do.

The first job was in the prison system. When they found I had worked with psychiatric patients, and had not been intimidated by them, they were sure I had skills they could use. It took some time to get cleared for the job. I guess they needed to be certain that I wasn't secretly some mobster's doll planning a sophisticated break out. After an extensive background check, finger prints, reference checks and repeated interviews, I went to work.

The job involved a fair amount of heavy lifting and pushing a heavy, unwieldy cart from cell to cell. At one of the facilities, I worked in several locations, and the cart had to be wheeled from building to building by going outside into the blistering sun or the howling wind and stinging, blowing sand. It didn't take long for me to realize that I wasn't strong enough and lacked the stamina to do the job properly. I will never do a job half-way, and I was thinking about running up the white flag. ED had taken me to the end of my physical resources.

God lead me to another job doing physicals for federal employees. It wasn't physically demanding, and I felt as though I had found my niche. I enjoyed the contact with the people, and I was in control of my little world. If I were in control, everything was a-okay. I was in the process of training a second woman to do the job when disaster struck.

On a hike earlier that year in Zion National Park, I twisted my ankle. It bugged me from time to time, but as with all symptoms personal, I ignored it. The pain intensified, and the leg began to throb. First, I tried the emergency department but they couldn't find the reason for the pain. It was rapidly becoming a living thing that gnawed at my leg twenty-four hours a day. Was I crazy, or was there something truly wrong with me. Since the medics couldn't find anything wrong, I was leaning toward crazy, but my leg still hurt like blazes.

When I tried the urgent care center, they x-rayed the leg and told me the films were negative. They prescribed a ten day course of antibiotics in case the inflammation had a septic origin. At the end of the medication, I was worse, so I went back to the center again, because I couldn't tolerate the pain any longer.

Unable to diagnose the problem, they sent me to the hospital to rule out phlebitis. When those tests proved negative, they told me to elevate the leg and see my family doctor. I couldn't get an appointment with him right away, and by the time I did, I was a basket case. When I finally saw him, he was quite alarmed and took another set of x-rays. Unable to diagnose my problem, he told me I should go to the Mayo Clinic in Scottsdale, Arizona.

At the Mayo Clinic, I was as frightened as I have ever been, and in as much pain as I have ever felt. Anyone who has ever experienced severe bone pain understands that the deep seated ache will simply not go away. The only way to get relief is through high powered drugs. For the first time in my life, I cried because of my own pain.

Do or Die Time

On day one, I had my first bone density test. My density was that of *a ninety year old woman*! They told me I had egg shell fragility of my bones. On the x-rays, my bones were ghostly casts, rather than the chalk white images of normal ones. Their nutritionist told me my calcium was dangerously low and started me on calcium supplements.

I'll say this for the Mayo Clinic. They are thorough. Every test known to mankind was performed on my failing body. The entire week it was test after test after test. Each one sent bolts of pain coursing through me, bringing tears to my eyes. The sad part of it was, I was angry with myself for showing weakness. Admitting to so much pain, and shedding tears made me nothing more than the member of the weaker sex my father always accused me of being.

When the test results came back, I felt vindicated. I had two fractures in my tibia, one in my fibula, several cracks in various vertebras and three or possibly four in my foot! The severe demineralization of my bones rendered the fractures invisible to conventional x-rays. My five weeks of whining in pain was justified. They put me in three casts for nearly six months and followed it with physical therapy.

After the first week, we went home for the weekend, then returned for a second week of tests. At least they had given me something for the pain. I was ashamed to have to take it but relieved that it helped my pain, and that I wasn't crazy. My next worry was addiction to the pain medication. Already fearful of alcohol abuse, I fretted about taking the very pills I so desperately needed.

It was a wake up call. For the first time, I understood how much trouble I was in. If I had known the physical damage I was doing to my body, would I have stopped? Would I have believed it was happening? I probably wouldn't have. The outside of me didn't look terminal or sick, or so ED told me. To my warped vision, I was a shinny red apple, but if you looked inside, I was rotting. Any mirror would have told me the truth, but I couldn't see it. My search for help began in earnest. It was time to do or die.

Back in Las Vegas, Monika, took me under her wing. We met at a time when both of us desperately needed something. We found each other and formed a friendship that will last a lifetime.

Monika is younger than I am, and an intelligent, outgoing woman from Germany with the traditional German will of iron. Over the next two years, she put tough love into practice. I wanted help, and I knew I couldn't do it alone. But I had to convince myself that God *could* do it. The concept that God could care about a fat, acne scarred sinner like me was beyond my grasp. I was thirsty for knowledge and searching for answers.

I needed the Truth fed to me one spoonful at a time, and the way Monika went about it was definitely God oriented. She spent hours with me and the Bible; preparing assignments for me to do and passages for study. Taking her time, she peeled God like an onion, one delicate layer at a time, each revealing more of His beauty to me. No one had ever spent so much time and energy loving me spiritually.

I knew I didn't deserve any of it. But, I am certain of one thing. If it had not been for those sessions with Monika, I would never have been able to understand God in the way I needed to in order to be healed. Those sessions literally *saved my life*.

My life during this period reminds me of an old joke. A terrible flood ravaged a community, and a rowboat came by and found an old farmer on the roof of his house.

"Come on; get in the boat, the water's still rising."

"No, I spent my whole life trusting in God, He'll save me."

In a few hours, a powerboat comes by to find the man on the peak of the roof.

"Come on; get in the boat, the water's still rising."

"No, I spent my whole life trusting in God, He'll save me."

Another hour passes and a helicopter finds the man clinging to his chimney as the muddy waters swirled higher. The helicopter crew threw down a lifeline.

"Come on; grab the line, the water's still rising. You're going to drown."

"No, I spent my whole life trusting in God, He'll save me."

The water covers the house and the man drowns. In heaven, he asks God, "Why didn't You save me. I spent my whole life worshiping You, and You let me die."

Glancing at his celestial clipboard, God said, "I sent you two boats and a helicopter, where were you?"

One of the first boats God sent me during my flood was my nutritionist, Joanie Gillespie. How was she going to help me? I hadn't eaten real food in decades. In her favor was the fact that after Mayo, I realized that if I wanted to go on living, I would have to eat. After much resistance, and constant badgering from Monika, I reluctantly agreed to see Joanie Gillespie.

In the beginning she saw me several times a week, and gave me a basic course in balanced nutrition. As a nurse, I had learned those things, but ignored my knowledge base over the years. She filled my head with nutrition facts. I trusted her from the beginning, and she spoon fed me, giving me only tasks she felt certain I would accomplish. It was important for me to succeed, and she knew it.

My first assignment was to drink water and go slowly, and she gave me hints on small frequent meals. Water was safe, I would drink it, and it put on no calories. She understood my knowledge base and hoped I would use it to develop the necessary emotional attachment to stay committed. I appreciate the fact that she never presses me or pushes me. Instead, she feeds me a steady stream of simply constructive encouragement. And, I can honestly say, I don't think I have ever met a more positive individual. Her bubbling, outgoing personality, tinged with the right amount of empathy and compassion is vocalized with the enthusiasm of a high school cheerleader. If all nutritionists were like this angel, the world would be a healthier place.

A second angel entered my life at nearly the same time. A friend at the Canyon Ridge Church suggested the name of a Christian counselor that she thought might be able to help me. After our unpleasant experience with Carolyn and her Christian counselor, the news struck Art like a rifle bullet. He categorically refused to let me go until he met the man. Following the meeting, we were both amazed at the peace, sincerity, empathy, and understanding we got from this gentle young man. His name is Chris Caldwell, and his training and credentials are impeccable.

On my first visit, I announced that I was a really tough cookie. He laughs about that now, but he got a fair picture from that statement of what he was up against. I entered therapy with one hand out for help and the other in front of my face to ward off the pain. Even through I wanted to change, the idea of giving up even a smidgen of control terrified me. I didn't realize that I wasn't in control. ED was. Chris was so wonderful that Art went with me a few times. It helped Chris understand our long and painful struggle.

With Chris' help, I realized that my identity was not with Art, or even with myself, but with Christ. He helped me understand that I was intent on being a victim. I had to be a victim of someone. In my childhood I was the victim of the dominant man in the house, and now, Art was the natural choice. Most of my married life, I had been trying to be what I thought Art wanted me to be. Since the input I received was garbled by my malfunctioning brain circuitry, I never felt I pleased anyone.

Chris showed me that my body was a gift from God, and that my behavior was desecrating God's temple. Despite that, it took me a long time to stop the desecration. I couldn't help myself; at least that's what ED made me believe.

When we discussed food, he questioned me about my eating habits when I was growing up. I told him about the comfort foods, spaghetti and other pastas, potatoes and breads. Now, I couldn't eat any of those foods. The thought of them made me physically ill. Was my revulsion of the food of my childhood another way I was trying to reject that childhood? I had never considered that before my sessions with Chris.

"What if I asked you to eat one strand of spaghetti?" Chris asked me one day.

It is hard to imagine how much that simple question terrified me. I broke out in a sweat and was unable to answer his question. I was terrified that it was a serious request. Then, I found out it was. His follow up question gave me pause as well.

"If you gained five pounds, would God still love you?"

Wrestling with these questions frustrated me so much; I thought I would lose my mind. I wanted to run away and hide. Thank God I didn't.

As my health deteriorated, God sent me healing angels too. Dr. Litchfield, a marvelous endocrinologist and my new internist, Dr. Schwartz, joined my health care team. Surrounded by all this angelic assistance, I continued to die.

When my leg finally healed, I received one of life's greatest gifts. I got a new daughter-in-law. In February of two thousand, David and Kathy were married in Arizona. Increasing the joy was the presence of the Bancroft Street bridge gang who came out *en mass* for the occasion.

David and Kathy chose a magnificent outdoor setting, with the rugged Arizona Mountains as a backdrop. Of course, Calvin, in his tux, and Tina, in her bridesmaid dress were in the wedding, and they made me so proud. It was absolutely perfect. But, as I stepped out to be seated before the kids came down the aisle, I felt that every eye in the wedding was on me, condemning me for my dress.

Four months earlier, Cal, Tina, Art and I met David and Kathy in Tucson, to be fitted with our tuxes and dresses. The girls worked on things for the reception, and we all had a great time. Both girls took me shopping for a dress. Believe me, they had a time finding one that fit my ravaged body. When they finally decided on the one I should wear, I was dumbfounded! I had never seen a dress like that one, and I was only the mother of the groom. It was way too fancy. People would think I was being grandiose or inappropriate.

Discovering the Monster Within

I could think of a dozen reasons why I shouldn't have that dress. I didn't deserve it. They wanted to hide my body. They were ashamed of me. It cost too much. None of that was true. My daughters by marriage loved me and were helping me celebrate. They wanted the day to be as special for me as it was for them. Still, it was hard for me to wear that dress. How sad. ED was able to take the kindness of my daughters-in-law and twist it into another cross for me to bear. They only wanted me to look and feel pretty, and the monster turned their love to a burden.

That night, at the reception, I was served a special meal. David and Kathy realized that I wouldn't eat the splendid dinner that they served, so they tried to give me something I would eat. My twisted perception received a dual message from this simple act of kindness. I was pleased and proud that they cared enough to do something so special for me, and at the same time, I was ashamed and humiliated that I had to eat it while others watched me. Knowing that I needed extra strength, my family and friends tried to subtly encourage me to eat. I was ashamed and humiliated, but not enough to change.

Back in Las Vegas, I landed a new job at the Montevista Psychiatric Hospital on the day shift. Two significant things occurred there that frightened me, and made me finally realize that ED was trying to kill me.

One day at work, I suddenly developed a large black spot in my visual field. As usual, I pretended it was nothing and tried to make light of it. But, it didn't go away, and I started to get nervous.

When I mentioned it to one of my colleagues, she became alarmed, and told me to call my doctor immediately. He referred me to an ophthalmologist and gave me her number. My anxiety increased when she told me she would see me that afternoon as an emergency.

At four o'clock, I saw her, and after the examination, she diagnosed a tear in the retina. She told me I would have to see a retinal specialist at once. It needed to be fixed before the tear worsened.

Within an hour, the retinal specialist saw me, and advised immediate laser surgery to seal the rent. He said he couldn't really fix it, but he could stop further damage. His therapy left me in such a state of shock that I never had time to be afraid of the surgery. All I could do was pray that God would spare my eyesight.

The worst part of the ordeal was trying to drive home wearing dark glasses with the setting sun shinning squarely in my eyes. I could hardly see a thing. Praying, I reminded God of the snowstorm on the way to my mom's and asked if He had one miracle left for me. He did. I still see spots before my eyes, but, after all, I am blond.

Next, I developed a hernia. I tried to ignore that, too. But, it wouldn't let me. When the surgeon repaired the hernia, he found my tissue as weak as wet toilet paper. He had to insert a mesh screen to hold things in place.

Frightened by my disintegrating body, I realized I had to do something, and soon. At Thanksgiving two years earlier, Kathy and David mentioned a place called Remuda Ranch, which dealt with in-depth therapy for persons with eating disorders. They did it in passing, without any pressure. Not ready for help, I relegated it to the back of my mind.

One day, while reading a Christian woman's magazine, I saw an advertisement for Ramuda Ranch, along with an eight hundred phone number. I was compelled to copy it down. Since a phone call would cost me nothing, why not? If you're gonna walk on water, you gotta get out of the boat. It was time to get out of the boat.

Over the next two days, I researched Remuda and talked to the people there as well as our insurance company. The price tag for the Remuda immersion therapy staggered me. And, the insurance company told me they wouldn't cover it. Disappointed, I dropped that idea immediately. I turned my attention to finding a good paying job and would use the money to find help in Las Vegas. That way, I wouldn't cost Art any more than I already had.

As a girl, I learned from my father that any money spent on women was wasted, and Art, was always worried about money. No matter how much we had, he wasn't comfortable with the amount. It was a constant source of anxiety for him. I couldn't possible spend any of it. Once more, I wanted something from someone that I felt they couldn't give me.

My sessions with Monika were becoming increasingly confrontational. Realizing that I was getting worse, she began to push me with all the Christian love she could muster.

"You like being a victim! You don't really want to get better!" she accused me.

Though I denied it, she made me think about it. I realized that she might be right, and the only way I could get better was if I wanted to. I did want too, didn't I?

At David's wedding, while our bridge group was having brunch, I told them that Art and I were thinking about a two-week train trip across Europe. We asked if any of them might want to go with us. The eight of us had taken any number of vacations together, and I hoped against hope some or all of them might join us. Jack Summers, who was retiring from his medical practice, and his wife Pat eagerly volunteered to go.

I didn't know at the time, but had one of them not agreed to go, Art would have killed the trip. The fact that Jack was a doctor gave Art the comfort he needed to agree to go. Art was so concerned about my health, he was afraid something awful might happen, and he would be alone in Europe with either a critically ill wife, or a corpse.

In August, the four of us set out on a wonderful adventure. I anticipated it so much, because everything would be new and different. I could relax and forget about food, broken bones, and detached retinas. My heart was heavy, and I was tired of being sick. Of course, food would be hard to ignore.

Things were different now. I was spending a great deal of time with God in prayer and worship. I opened my heart to my angels and felt I was starting to make progress. Joanie helped me prepare nutritionally as much as I would let her. She reiterated the need to keep my nutrition balanced. I took soy nuts, protein bars, dried fruits and things I knew I would eat. There would be an abundance of delicious foods in the countries we visited to balance my diet, but I knew I wouldn't eat them. ED had convinced me that my nuts and berries were therapy enough.

Another problem was my attention span. I had progressively more and more trouble staying focused, and it frightened me. I firmly believe that I had starved my brain to the point that its circuits were malfunctioning.

From the beginning, my dream vacation became an approach avoidance conflict. I couldn't wait to go, but I was ashamed that I wasn't strong enough to carry a single piece of luggage. When my bones were broken, Art lugged me around in a wheelchair and took over the household chores I had done for years. Here was another thing I couldn't do.

When I saw Jack and Pat's smiling faces at the Cincinnati airport, I felt a surge of relief. If anything happened, I was among friends. Art wasn't the only one with insecurities. It didn't hurt that Jack was a doctor.

I was determined to keep up with everyone. To do so, I had to eat more. So, at the beginning, I worked hard at eating. Fortified with nuts and bars, I felt I could do it.

The trip started in London. After a full day of sight seeing, the four of us went to dinner together. I avoided sauces, gravies and sweets, like the plague, but did eat some protein and used my additives.

Art is a train nut. He loves trains of all kinds, and a day trip on the Orient Express was to be the highlight of the London segment. Unfortunately, Art got food poisoning at an Italian restaurant in London the night before and was greener than the conductor's uniforms when we boarded the historic coach, Persus, for the two-hour trip to Folkstone Harbor.

Ours was the royal coach used by Winston Churchill, among others. It had its own separate dining compartment for four people in the center of the car. We were assigned to the enclosure. When I glimpsed the table service, my heart started to pound. Lace table cloths covered the table and an assortment of silver cutlery and glassware portended a major feast. I proved to be a prophet.

Discovering the Monster Within

Starting with bottles of Champagne and Claret, we were served munchies of Calamata olives and assorted nuts. Lunch consisted of cream of asparagus soup, Guinea fowl with sage dressing, carrots and snap peas. Dessert was a mélange of raspberries and blueberries.

I was able to pick my way through lunch by eating bits of each thing, picking at the food and eating only what was absolutely safe. The high tea served on the way back was harder to fake. Finger sandwiches, country scones, strawberries and cream with jam and a selection of cakes left me with nothing to eat. I did enjoy the tea from Ceylon and China.

With a magical setting, food to die for, surrounded by friends and the man I love, I missed half of the adventure of a lifetime, as ED's icy fingers strangled me with fear. How sad.

The train whisked us to the romantic city of Paris. A whirl of activity and sightseeing left me near exhaustion half way through each day. I must have used the calories from the wine I drank to give me the energy to go on, because though I ate food, it was not enough.

One night in Paris, we went to the Neurvo Eve Nightclub. It was a classic French follies show, complete with bare breasts, long legged dancers, comedians, trapezes and another wonderful meal. I did venture to eat the pate, when I was assured that it was all meat, and it *was* wonderful. Yes, the richness of it made me feel guilty, but I was in no position to purge. The guilt nearly suffocated me.

As we moved on to Switzerland, my anxiety levels increased. Monika was back in her native Germany, and was coming to Zermat to meet us. The meal they planned for us that first night was a magnificent pork roast stuffed with whole prunes. Served plain, with only its juices, it was delicious, and I surprised myself by eating the whole serving.

The meeting with Monika went without a hitch, and I fooled myself into thinking I impressed everyone with my new appetite, except ED of course. Leaving Zermat on the Glacier Express, we went through the most spectacular Alpine scenery on the planet before arriving in Italy. Excited as I was, the fatigue of the trip settled in. With no energy reserves left, I found myself fighting to stay awake at the slightest lull.

Italy was an eating disaster from the get go. First, pasta, and second I knew the trip was nearly over. I could survive on salads and soy nuts. Fortunately, Jack coaxed me into trying *Insalata Caprice*, a combination of fresh tomatoes, basil and fresh Buffalo mozzarella cheese that proved to be a Godsend. The only dressing was the basil, so I ate it all. I loved it, and it became the staple of my Italian diet.

As tired and malnourished as I was, I pushed myself to keep going. On our last full day in Rome, we visited the Coliseum. A merciless August sun turned the arena into a cauldron. At the end of the tour, our guide told us we could climb a steep flight of stone stairs up four stories to look out over the arena from where the aristocracy sat. Jack's wife Pat was wilted like a thirsty violet, but Jack, the intrepid photographer, started up, and I followed him. Art took the day off, still feeling ill from the earlier case of food poisoning. On the climb, I noticed Jack kept a weather eye on me, but somehow I made it to the top.

It was a spectacular view of the patch of earth where so many men, women and even children, many of them Christians, suffered horrible deaths. I had a lot in common with them. A rampaging animal was trying to eat me alive, too, but mine was inside my head.

That last night in Rome, Art was too tired to go out for dinner, so Jack took his wife Pat, a wonderful woman from Florida named Roz, whom we met on the trip, and me for a walk and dinner on the Via Veneto. As we sat at the romantic sidewalk café, I felt sad that I couldn't relax and enjoy the table the way my friends did. Oh, I put up a good front, but it was simply another meal, another stress, and another temptation to lose control. I don't know why I was so up tight. ED would never allow that to happen.

When I returned to Las Vegas, I found I had better luck with breakfast and lunch than I did supper. I could justify the calories at those two meals as necessary, and I could easily work them off. That's another trick anorexics use. I know one gal who has a computer program. She scrupulously watches her calories and enters them into the program. It calculates exactly the amount of exercise needed to work off the calories, and she does.

Supper was harder. I couldn't get over the habit of eating dinner, picking at the leftovers and then purging. I figured if I wasn't exercising, I wasn't burning up any calories. There was no way I could go to sleep on all those calories.

My weight continued to drop, and with everything else going on, the doctors who were looking after me started pushing for tube feedings, which I adamantly refused.

I continued counseling with Chris, and slowly came to the conclusion that my behavior was a form of blasphemy. I was telling God that He made a mistake with me. The temple God had given me wasn't suitable, so I was remodeling it. God loved me, and I was making God sad. It was time to do something about that.

For the next couple of months, I tried the insurance company again, but got nowhere. Monika hung in there with me, gradually turning up the heat. Joanie knew my turmoil, as did Chris, and their loving support nudged me in the right direction. Coupled with my deteriorating body, it all came together.

The choice was mine. It was time to decide not only if I wanted to live, but to determine the quality the remainder of my life would have. God had provided me with the help I needed. He opened my eyes to the monster. It was my turn to help. To realize that I was in control of that decision made me determined to get help. Still, the money issue haunted me. If the insurance wouldn't cover it, where would I get the money?

Mistakenly, I picked Monika's shoulder to cry on. What a wonderful mistake that proved to be. Confiding in her about Remuda, I told her I couldn't spend Art's money like that. Monika, who was getting more anxious about my condition, *exploded*.

"Pat, I don't want to hear any more of that! I've heard enough! You don't want to get better; all you want to do is make excuses! That money is half yours, and you deserve to use it any way you see fit, especially if it will save your life! Go on; deny God some more! You like the victim role. You like being sick!" Then, with tears in her eyes, she hugged me and prayed with me.

After she was gone, I spent time on my knees with God. It was as if I had been struck by lightening. She was right! It *was* partly my money, and I needed to use it if I was going to live.

Christmas two thousand was rapidly approaching, and the boys were coming with their wives. Carolyn weighed heavily on my mind, and I longed to see her, too. But, I knew that would never be. Despite my new resolve, my heart was in my throat as I approached Art with my ideas. I told him more about Remuda, the cost, and my desire to get help and to go on living. Trying to read his emotions in his expression, I assumed the worst and immediately reassured him that it would be all right if he said, no.

My dear mate's eyes filled with tears of joy and relief. The moment was so overwhelming it took the breath I had been holding completely away. He was willing to do it, *for me*! Sadly, he would have done it anytime I would have asked him to over the past forty years. Failing to realize that I was a person worthy of that kind of love robbed us both of half-a-lifetime of happiness and health. Money wasn't the issue. He'd get it anyway he had to. Since I was down to eighty-two pounds, he was afraid I might die before he could get me help.

When the kids came, I gave them the literature and information packet from Remuda. After they read it, we watched the informational video included in the packet. The joy on their faces sent shivers through me, as they hugged me and offered words of encouragement. Years of worrying about me starving myself to death might finally be ending. Their expressions carried an equal measure of relief. They were so excited they wanted me to get on the phone immediately and call Remuda.

Early in January, I called for an appointment. There is usually a long waiting list, but when they heard my story, they gave me an appointment for later that month.

Discovering the Monster Within

How did I feel? Relieved, frightened, anxious and humbled by the love of God and of my family and friends, my emotions were in overdrive. I packed, cried, prayed, and cried some more as I prepared my things for Remuda. And I was able to suppress the maniacal screams of ED, as he tried to claw his way into my consciousness.

CHAPTER 12

How did I Get Here?

How did my life end up such a mess? Although I must take most of the credit, I didn't get here alone. Society was a great help. Its attitude toward body image is one of ED's staunchest allies. Everywhere we look, thin is in.

This attitude is best epitomized by the popular TV series Allie Mc-Beal, staring Calista Flockhart. Although she has openly denied being anorexic, Ms. Flockhart has the body build to be an anorexic poster girl. On the show, she is the lead character surrounded by voluptuous females like, Courtney Thrown-Smith, Lucy Liu, Portia deRossi and Jane Krakowski. Despite that, every male on the show ignores them to go after the scarecrow. The message, thin is where it's at.

Anyone who has turned on a TV set in the past year know who Jared, the Subway boy is. Although the young man had an overeating problem, he now fits the all-American profile of thin, thanks to Subway's low-fat sandwiches.

Popular Hollywood star Reneé Zelwigger was the subject of multiple media articles concerning her role in an upcoming movie called "Bridget." To successfully portray the character, Ms. Zelwigger had to balloon up to an enormous one hundred thirty pounds. To ease the pain of becoming the national blimp, she was paid an unreasonable amount of money for each of these disgraceful pounds. At that weight, she is still a beautiful woman, but not to our thin-is-in society.

I would be the first to agree that many Americans weigh too much. But, we are a diet crazy society, and that is a major building block in the construction of an eating disorder. In a study done by Crisp and Burney on anorexic men, they found that prior to the onset of disease the majority of the men were overweight and had dieted.

According to the National Association of Anorexia Nervosa, adolescents who were categorized as severe dieters had an eighteen times higher chance of developing an eating disorder than did their peers. Those considered moderate dieters developed the disease five times more often than those who ate normally.

Dieting among the younger generation, whose role model is Brittany Spears, is practiced at an alarming rate. Teen magazines are replete with aesthetic looking young women who look like they could use a good meal. Thin is in.

Silence is another companion of the disease. Since I have begun to talk openly about my disease, numerous individuals have told me about a friend, family member, relative or acquaintance that they believe is anorexic. They talk about it to me, but not to the individual with the problem. When I ask why, the answer is always the same. "I don't know how to go about it." I understand; my family and friends went through the same thing.

Public school heath classes discuss the nutritional aspects of food; warn against the dangers of high fat and fast food diets and addictive behavior. Excessive eating or anorexic behaviors are seldom or never mentioned.

An equal indictment could be delivered to the medical profession. Physicians are poorly equipped to handle eating disorders. Medical school supplies little to no information concerning nutrition, or how to recognize and treat ED. Rather than broaching the subject with the patient and getting the appropriate nutritional and psychiatric assistance, the disease is most often ignored. I believe the incidence of anorexia is grossly underreported.

Despite the societal assistance, I can't blame it for everything. Most of it was my own, self-destructive behavior. The faulty tapes in my head had convinced me that I should suffer. I deserved nothing. I should never have been born and deserved to die. I didn't belong anywhere, because I didn't do enough to earn a place.

Most importantly, those tapes convinced me that food was my enemy. Hunger was strength. Tasting food was the same as eating it. Besides, I might like it. Scales and measuring tapes became who I was. If I gain an ounce, I've failed. One bit of food would put weight on a body that was already grotesquely fat.

I was also able to stop my ears to the fear and frustration of family and friends who couldn't understand how I could do this to myself. They couldn't understand why I simply couldn't sit down at the table and eat. I could never explain my fear to them. I was so afraid of eating; I would rather die than gain an ounce. You can't say that to someone you love, but I showed it by my behavior every day.

None of those things were ever on a conscious level until now. I was consumed by fear of my mortal enemy, food. The result of that fear was a constant level of depression, obsessive-compulsive behavior and victimization. Thanks to my early training, I rationalized my way out of it. Any self-respecting person with ED can rationalize their way *out of anything*, and I was a professional in that art.

I have an addictive personality with obsessive overtones. Unlike an addiction to alcohol, where the alcohol becomes the problem, with ED, the addiction is not to the food, but to the behavior as expressed in the familiar binge-purge or anxiety-restriction cycles.

Consider how an addiction works. Ingesting an addicting substance has two possible effects. It dulls the senses easing the psychic pain that caused the addiction, and alleviates the physical symptoms of withdrawal. The effect is loss of control, as the individual can no longer control the amounts of the addictive they need. As the addiction worsens, more of the addicting substance is needed to get the same effect. ED and its vicious cycle work exactly the same way.

Another of my addictions was to laxatives, and I took so many over the years that I became definitely addicted to them. Getting my paralyzed bowel to even gurgle without their help caused major withdrawal symptoms. Half my time at Remuda was spent in gas cramp nirvana.

I was also habituated to alcohol, and it took me sometime to admit that to myself. Considering my father's problems, I wonder how I ever allowed it to sneak up on me. After much introspection, I think I know. In the last few years before Remuda, I began to drink more than I should. My body was starving; my brain was starving, and my soul was starving. Still, I refused to nourish any part of me. I think my subconscious realized that alcohol was a source of calories and craved it for the energy I needed. But, those kinds of calories never helped my underlying malnutrition.

The real reason I drank was as old as the history of alcohol itself. My health was in shambles; my daughter was gone; my husband was drifting away, and I couldn't see any way to alter the outcome. I drank to ease the pain, and it worked. It also fit my compulsive personality. From personal hygiene, to dress, to housekeeping, to nagging at the kids and Art, I was a compulsive perfectionist. It wasn't a large leap to compulsiveness with alcohol.

Besides the pain relief, alcohol had another positive effect for me, even if it was a negative for everyone around me. It loosened my tongue. The pent up hostilities that I had harbored so long escaped their confinement to surface at the tip of my tongue.

Fortunately, I never reached the stage my father did. I never became truly addicted. When the majority of the pain left my life after Remuda, it was possible for me to control my intake of alcohol. I do not avoid alcohol; I just make sure my social drinking is controlled.

Obsession became a way of life, even in my thought processes. For example, I see a French fry. It triggers this obsessive loop: French fry = calories = gross can't stand that = stomach = fat = fear = avoidance.

How did I Get Here?

It blinks through my mind in a subconscious millisecond when I eat anything but lettuce.

How did I begin to break a cycle so vicious? How did I gain the courage to come to Remuda? First, I had to determine if anything in my life was more important than not eating. Then, I decided I wanted to live and not die. Sounds so obvious, but with ED as a houseguest, you die so slowly you don't realize you're doing it.

In the concentration camp at Auschwitz, they had a starvation cell in the prison barracks. People were locked in that cell without food until they died. Some of them were able to live weeks without food before the inevitable. Their symptoms were cardinal and rapid. I gave myself just enough food to not die, and I did it for years. It was time to change that. I wasn't ready to die. When I looked at my quality of life, there wasn't any quality in it.

To change, I had to admit two things that were not easy. First, I had a potentially fatal disease. Second, I could do nothing about it myself. I needed help!

Because it's so vital to the understanding of ED, it's important to reiterate that eating disorders are control issues. The most difficult thing for an anorexic to do is relinquish control of the only thing in their lives they feel they *can* control. Rose Memo, a therapist who deals with eating disorders on a daily basis, feels that many anorexics find it easier to relinquish control to God than to another human being, like a therapist. In her experience, she notes that those clients who get a firm grasp on "the God piece," will be the ones who recover.

I have been a religious person since mom began taking us to church when I was a teen. Had anyone asked me, I would have identified myself as a Christian. I attended church regularly, was involved in many of the activities of the church, and could tell you a great deal about God. But, like so many Christians, it was only lip service for most of my life, because though I knew God intellectually, I never accepted His power in my life.

Discovering the Monster Within

There were a number of times in my life, when God took a direct hand in events. The snowstorm on the way to my mothers and getting me home after my detached retina surgery were two of them. I saw the miracles; was the direct beneficiary of their power, but still didn't understand God's love for me.

Like all of us, there were times in my life when I wondered where God was. Where was He when my daughter's head was filling with lies? Where was He when Dennis was born? Where was He when my marriage was falling apart? The answer is simple. He was right there, where He always is.

The two years before I went to Remuda, I was like Jonah. God gave Jonah a job to do, and instead of doing it he ran. Leaping on a ship he was determined to run to the ends of the earth so God couldn't find him. God did, and Jonah's plight as a temporary snack for a great fish is history. Like the prophet, I tried to run from God by hiding behind my insecurity. But, God wouldn't let go. He kept pushing me gently in the right direction until I saw the light.

I'm not sure exactly how it happened, or when it happened. I know my councilor, Chris, my nutritionist Joanie, and my friend Monika were all responsible for bringing me God's message in their own way. They plowed the field and planted the seeds so the therapists at Remuda could reap the harvest.

What was the startling revelation that changed my life? It was the simple realization that God loved me. He loved me for myself, not for anything I ever did for Him. It was the hardest truth I ever had to accept. All my life, I felt worthless. From the Archer family to the Burkley family I felt I had to earn my way. I had to give, give, give; do, do, do. I had to prove to everyone that I belonged. I didn't have to do that with God. I couldn't do it without the love of God.

As I studied the Bible, and discussed passages with Monika, I gradually became aware that God loved me, even if I didn't love myself. And, He always had. One simple verse says it all.

1 John 4:19 "We love him, because he first loved us."

How did I Get Here?

Another inescapable conclusion had to be drawn. My behavior was directly accusing God of making a mistake. I was telling Him that the body he had given me had design flaws. It was too big. I knew better how it should be. I was making it a fit vessel. That couldn't be. God doesn't make mistakes. I remember seeing a child's T-shirt with a mournful little urchin on the front. Beneath it were the words, "God don't make no junk." No, He doesn't. Even though I was trying to tell Him He had.

These simple words became my halcyon cry in recovery. God doesn't make mistakes. I've placed everything in my life in His hands. Sink or swim, I'm on God's team.

The other thing that helped me was making God a *meaningful* part of my daily life. I have come to know God as I would a personal friend. I talk to Him multiple times a day, both formally and informally. I ask His advice, direction and guidance. Most often, I ask for His help. And, my prayers are always answered, even when the answer is no.

I would be the last to imply that God is the only solution that leads to a cure for anorexia. It isn't. There are countless examples of cures where God has not been mentioned. These people found other ways to free themselves of their monsters. But, in each case, they had to relinquish the control of their lives to a therapist. Mine happened to be God.

Once I latched onto "the God piece," my decision to pursue therapy crystallized. What better person to relinquish control to than God? He loved me while I denied Him; forgave me for trying to tell Him He made a mistake, and constantly sent His human angels to nudge me toward the therapy that would save my life. Thank you, God. I owe You.

CHAPTER 13

The House of Judah

My House of Judah, The Remuda Treatment Center for Adult Female Eating Disorders is a professional, Biblically-based, non-denominational program exclusively related to the treatment of adult and adolescent females with eating disorders. Since I had given control of my life to God, and He was now dictating my actions, that were important to me.

The Remuda staff recognizes that eating disorders are not diseases, rather the prime symptom of a monster with many tentacles insinuating deep underlying events, patterns, cultural pressures and family responsibilities that are dysfunctional. Identifying, understanding and coping with these distinctive feelings and behaviors are the targets of the sixty-day immersion therapy at their facilities. And, they do it in a warm, non-threatening therapeutic environment where one can work to resolve their individual conflicts. I think their mission statement best sums this up.

"We want to remain a Christian island of hope for those courageous enough to reach out for help. Our mission is to provide:

1. A non-denominational Biblically-based scripture emphasis.

2. Safe and secure healing environment providing broad ranged therapeutic activities.
3. A system that is grounded in a constant philosophy of individualized treatment throughout the continuum of care.
4. Opportunities for family involvement leading to a recognition of the emotional impact of the eating disorder on the entire family structure, educating and training the family in healthy styles of communication and interaction.
5. Programs dedicated to being about a continuing life-style change, encouraging self-trust and confidence so that life may be fully embraced, released from the pain of obsessions, compulsions and addictions.
6. A gently, yet challenging therapeutic environment with an entire staff committed to meeting the medical, nutritional, psychological and spiritual needs of our clients and patients.
7. Ongoing supportive relationships helping to ensure continuing recovery so that lives are no longer ruled by food or fear.
8. Growing relationships with allied health professionals worldwide.

Over the next two months, these lofty principles would be my life and they wasted no time getting us into the swing of things.

For someone who has survived half-a-lifetime on the daily caloric equivalent of a handful of butterfly wings and a couple of spider webs, it seemed to me as if all we did was eat all day long. Certain foods were considered required, and if we did not eat them, supplements equivalent to the missed calories were administered. Those who refused the supplement were deemed uncooperative, and if that became a pattern was reason for discharge from the program. We were served breakfast, a ten a.m. snack, lunch, a three p.m. snack, supper and a bed time snack. It was the classic diabetic diet pattern used to flatten insulin response.

Only once did I not eat my required portions. I didn't put dressing on my salad, and had to take the supplement. I used salad dressing the rest of the time I was there. After all, I was spending a lot of money to be here, and I wasn't going to waste it. I was determined to eat everything they gave me. I wanted to get well! I *had* to get well. To prove it to myself, the first night at Remuda, I ate my first dessert in three decades.

To be certain the bulimic's among us didn't exercise our inalienable rights to puke up a perfectly fine meal, we were required to stay at the table for half-an-hour. When asked about this repulsive behavior, most bulimics will politely say, "I lost my meal." That's my style, too. Maybe if we called it what it is, it would remove some of the romance from the behavior. A monitor joined us for each meal to insure compliance. If an emergency bath-room run was required, one of the staff went too. We were not allowed to flush the John until they inspected the toilet bowl for contraband. That's what I call a *dedicated* professional.

Some of my fellow soldiers learned creative and disgusting ways not to eat. They would hide food in their baggy sleeves and deposit it in secluded portions of the property. Another revolting trick was to vomit food into clothing, say a sweater they were carrying. Then they would roll it up so the offending cargo couldn't be spotted. Later, they washed out the odoriferous garment and reused it.

Many of the girls were so nutritionally challenged that tube feeding was required to sustain them. One of these creative children learned how to siphon her nighttime tube feeding into a spare cup that could be hidden in a drawer until the coast was clear. Then, she dumped it out the window.

Exercise was another trick some girls tried to keep from gaining weight. Although unsupervised exercise was forbidden, one girl would wait until lights out to begin a rigorous exercise routine aimed at working off every excess calorie she had taken in. It placed a tremendous strain on her roommate, who was torn between turning her in and letting her continue to destroy the effects of the therapy. The exerciser was eventually asked to leave. Some of the others were more subtle and got away with it.

The House of Judah

As with the first day, each day began with a weigh-in to check the success or failure of the treatment plan. They knew exactly how much weight each of us should gain, depending on our state of nutrition when we arrived. Although most of us slept in our own nightclothes, they provided us with a standard gown. These gowns were the only things worn at the weigh in. And, since we all obsessed about our weight, we were never told the number until the last day at the ranch. One of the valuable lessons I learned early on was that the scale was your enemy. The scale is to the anorexic or bulimic as the shot of whiskey is to the alcoholic. One step onto a scale is falling off the wagon.

Each day, the next day's menus were presented to us. We were allowed to choose what we wanted to eat. Everyone received the same sized portions, and we knew that whatever we chose, we would be required to eat all of it. I thought of Linda and her peas!

Two days into the program, I committed my first grave error. Conversation at the table was encouraged, but food as a subject was forbidden. That particular day the choices were finger sandwiches on either bread or crescent rolls. Remembering the greasy feel of a crescent roll, I had chosen the bread option. Without thinking, I said, "Thank God I didn't order the crescent roll. I don't think I could have gotten that down."

To my horror, the girl sitting next to me was about to take a bite of her crescent roll sandwich. Without a word, she dropped it onto her plate, pushed back her chair and fled the dinning hall. Entirely focused on my needs, my problems, and myself, I had unintentionally and unnecessarily hurt her. Had there been a hole there, I would have crawled into it and gladly covered myself with dirt.

That made me realize that there were others here struggling as much as I was, and for all of us it was a matter of life and death. None of us wanted to be here, and I had just injured another warrior in the battle for survival. That night, I prayed that God, and the woman, would forgive me for my insensitivity and selfishness. It took nearly two weeks before she realized how repentant a sinner I was, and how awful the episode made me feel. When she did, God answered my prayer, and she forgave me. Not only did she forgive me, but became one of my best friends at Remuda. That was a tough lesson for me to learn.

Another problem surfaced at once. Cut off from my laxative supply, I had to learn to have my own, unassisted bowel movements. That was a chore. Constipation and cramping became a daily trial. Still, I tried, because if I couldn't retrain them, other horrors awaited.

My weight didn't respond as the nutritionist desired, and they held a summit conference to decide if I needed tube feedings, supplements or bigger snacks. Ever since those bozos in Las Vegas first mentioned tube feedings, I vigorously opposed them, and could see no earthly reason to change my opinion now. Fortunately, a booster orange drink was prescribed rather than the less desirable options.

If we did not eat everything we were supposed too, liquid supplements replaced the missing calories. When the going got tough, and ED had nearly convinced me to not only refuse the food, but the supplement too, I convinced myself that food was a medication. It was the treatment for my particular kind of disease. As with anyone who suffers from a potentially fatal illness, if I wanted to live, I had to undergo the therapy.

It was strange. With all my nursing background and nutritional education, I never considered salad dressing a food. That's why it was so easy for me to pass it up on that one occasion. As far as I was concerned, it had no redeeming social value. My pea-sized brain didn't compute the fat calories it contained. It also ignored the fact that if a diet had no fat in it, the body burned protein for fuel. No wonder I looked like a starving imitation of a rail-thin fashion model. I was literally cannibalizing my own muscles to stay alive.

At the end of the second week of the program, God had given me the courage to write to all the children, including Carolyn, and to my little brother to tell him of my situation. Included in each of the children's letters was the official invitation to family week. The act of pouring my love into each of those letters took a great load from my mind, and allowed me to focus even more on my therapy sessions.

Besides my reluctant bowels, I developed another bothersome set of symptoms. Intense night sweats plagued me. I was certain I was experiencing a form of alcohol withdrawal. Convinced that this proved I was an alcoholic, I was too ashamed to mention the symptoms to my fellow combatants or our angels.

To my relief, I discovered all of us were sweating like a gaggle of old maids at an AARP convention awaiting an overdue shipment of Premarin. The explanation came in nutrition class. Our bodies were being fed sufficient calories for the first time in years, and our metabolism was increasing from what our starved bodies felt was an unlimited supply of fuel. I visualized Pac Man, from one of the original video games. He became my body gobbling up the calories it had been deprived of for a lifetime.

Unable to get my balky bowels to respond, I had absolutely no natural peristalsis left thanks to the years of laxative abuse. I tried everything they had to safely reinstitute nature. They even did an ultrasound to rule out gallbladder obstruction. Fortunately there were no problems there.

Once they knew it wouldn't kill me, they dumped 1000 c.c. of Go Lightly, a liquid with the gastronomic appeal of flavored chalk, into my depleted, dehydrated system. It worked for a time, but things gradually slowed again. After the appropriate waiting period, they dosed me a second time. The pain and cramping were so severe I wanted to cry, but I didn't. I didn't cry about much of anything.

As time went on, I became frightened that I was here, doing all these things and wasn't feeling anything yet. The only emotions I could feel were the shame and self-loathing I brought with me. I was still too detached from the process.

Five days per week we had chapel, provided by various guest pastors, ranch staff, or special guests. I found those times an inspirational way to begin the day. The messages were non-denominational and applicable to the trials and tribulations of life at the ranch. Prayer was an important part of every day for the program and for me personally.

The group therapy process was the main vector for exploring the thoughts feelings and relationship issues that allowed the monster to control our lives. Another purpose of group therapy is to encourage you to face your feelings and issues as you discover them and get feedback from others about them. The discussions were guided away from eating disorders, which was only a symptom, to the real issues that caused the symptoms. Home Group, as our primary group therapy unit was called, allowed us to learn relationship skills that could be used in real-life-situations.

My group had six other women in it, and it reminded me of my father's old Alcoholic's Anonymous groups, absent the dance afterward. The analogy made me uncomfortable at first, particularly since I secretly believed that I might be an alcoholic. I didn't know if I should stand up and say, "Hi, I'm Pat and I'm an alcoholic," or, "Hi my name's Pat and I'm an anorexic, bulimic basket case!" It didn't matter. It seemed that I was uncomfortable about nearly everything.

In this group, I developed some of my most positive and negative relationships. One of the other girls had a problem with chewing her fingernails. Chewed to the quick, they threatened to bleed spontaneously at any moment. She asked us to help her with her problem. It had become second nature, and she didn't even know when she was doing it. If we saw her biting her nails, she asked us to remind her she was doing it.

Those of us on medications had to line up to be dosed. Waiting for my daily calcium fix, she stood in the line ahead of me. Assuming she was earnest about her request, I quietly touched her on the elbow, reminded her of her request and told her that she was biting her nails. I felt I had done what she wanted me to do.

I have been many things in my life, some of which I am ashamed of. One of my admirable characteristics is an absolute lack of guile. I made the mistake of thinking she was that way, too. At Home Group the next day, I was in for a major league surprise.

She stood up in the session and informed the others that I was trying to take over the group. I was dominating, and invading her space. I was an unconscionable eavesdropper who was intrusive with the other girls, and she wanted me to know that it wasn't appreciated. "Everyone is talking about you," she concluded.

Stunned, I sat there with my mouth open. I was so shocked, and speechless I didn't even try to defend myself. Flushing, I could feel the heat rise in my face. Then, something happened that should have shown me how dysfunctional my emotions were. Shame enveloped me like a shroud, and I felt certain that I had done some terrible thing. I skulked from the session as a felon flees a crime scene. In the weeks ahead, I was able to understand that her rage and the attack on me were her communication problems and not mine. Still, it didn't help me that day.

Another exercise at Remuda requires us to write to our family members and ask them what my eating disorder had done to each of them and ask for their forgiveness. Shortly after Home Group, I stopped by the mailbox. Art's response to my letter was there. As I read the damage I had done to my beloved partner it was almost more than I could bear. On top of the girl's attack, it made it one of the worst days I spent at Remuda.

Three days later, she attacked me in Home Group again. Fortunately, I had an appointment with the psychiatrist shortly afterwards. Psychotherapy is a routine part of the treatment protocol at Remuda, and believe me, all of us needed it. Surprised that I found my tears, I began to cry. I told him the whole story.

"Pat, you still don't understand that everything is not about you. It's about her, not you. Everything in your life is not about you. When things don't turn out the way you expect them to, it's not always due to something you did or didn't do," he told me gently.

Once again me, me, me, always me was in the way. Still, I couldn't let it go. She had accused me of taking over every group I was in, and I knew in my heart that wasn't true, but my head didn't know it. I had to test it for myself.

Each of us was in a number of specialty groups, besides Home Group, tailored to specific problems in one's life. Groups like Anxiety, Women's Issues, Trauma and Loss fit many of us. Nail-biter and I shared Alcohol Abuse, Sexual Abuse and Bulimic groups, as well as Obsessive Compulsive Behaviors. Maybe she disliked me because we were so much alike.

Approaching every group leader, I told them of her indictments and asked the validity of her charges. If they thought they were true, I begged them to help me to change. Every one of them looked at me aghast and told me her charges were absolutely false.

"You're a joy Pat. We admire you, and we're glad you're here. You can't make everyone else's problems your own," they said. "It's not about you. It's her problem."

Finally, it got through to me, and my head and my heart were in agreement. The episode taught me that important lesson. In my heart, I knew I had done no wrong. But the faulty program on the tape in my head that ED ran for me wouldn't let my brain acknowledge it. That was the secret. Face the problem. Recognize the error on the tape. Erase it, and fix it.

Occasionally, the girls at the ranch did things that were too much for even the angels who cared for us. One poor child had amphetamines smuggled into her by a first class enabler, so she could counteract the effects of the added calories. When that wasn't enough, she waited until lights out and began a rigorous exercise program in her room to finish the job. It only proved that those who embrace the monster will go to any length to protect him and feed his hunger.

A new girl was admitted to the ranch and things began to disappear. She was backward in table manners, speech and dress. Unfortunately, she was forward and intrusive in almost everything else. That's the last thing a person with an eating disorder can tolerate. Some of the girls accused the new girl of the escalating thefts.

The House of Judah

One morning, unannounced, the staff told us we would spend the day in the chapel while our rooms were searched. Each of us could accompany the search party when our room came up. When the search was completed, the staff brought us back to the chapel.

As the morning dragged on, the tension escalated to unbearable levels. When you place twenty insecure, self-conscious women with ED in a confined space, the tension is generated by the mere apposition of bodies and the situation becomes volatile in a hurry.

Finally, the search was over and they released us. The new girl was asked to leave and the burglaries ceased. My heart was heavy as I watched her go. Everyone with ED needs help, and reaches out for life. Had she declined to do so and reached out for death instead? Had she been forced to come here, and this was her way out?

Despite it all, I had an unsettling thought. The other girls in her Home Group clique despised her for her slovenly manners, dress and speech. Could one of them have been the thief and framed the helpless girl? Could they have done it to pressure the ranch into sending her home? I hope not, but as I watched the reactions of the other girls I couldn't really be sure.

Art's first visit was an emotional one, and we held each other and celebrated with tears of joy. At last someone was doing something about the greatest source of Art's anxiety, and on both counts that someone was me! He helped me choose cards to write to David and Kathy whose first anniversary was imminent. It was hard to let him go to start the trip back home.

In our spare time, we were encouraged to color in coloring books, paint, draw or otherwise express our artistic talents. Feeling the simple joy of the child inside me, I scribbled. Not blessed with artistic talent that would make Rembrandt nervous, I decided to keep a diary. That night, I wrote, "David and Kathy married a year, and I am healing. What will next February bring?" More content than I had been in days; I toddled off to my cot and slept like a baby.

Discovering the Monster Within

An interesting facet of the Remuda experience is their experiential therapies. They include Equine Activities, Aquatic Play (weather permitting) Psychodrama, Nutritional Food Challenges, One Sense Walks and Self Image Experiences.

Due to my eggshell bones, anything halfway physical was scratched from my agenda. This included riding the horses in the Equine Activity. One fall from a horse could be fatal to me. I did participate in the rest of the activity and grooming the magnificent animals was a true joy.

The Equine Activity was an exercise in communication. It taught us to emphasize and embrace the abilities that each of us have and use them to care for and grow in a relationship, this time with a horse. Because he was a horse, when I spoke to him, he didn't always hear or understand what I said to him. Those of us with the monster are the same way. We don't hear, and when we do, what we hear frequently isn't what was said. Working with the horse helped me to understand that.

Plus, the only horses I had ever been close to was over our neighbor's fence when I was a child. I had no idea what I was doing. I made mistakes over and over before I asked for help. That taught me that I needed help, and it was okay to ask for it. The equestrian staff helped me understand that I couldn't be perfect, and didn't have to be. God never expected it of me. Why should I expect it of myself?

Another interesting exercise was the One Sense Walk. We had to take a walk around the property and concentrate on only one sense. If that were hearing, then sight, touch and smell were masked. As I toured the now familiar grounds with all but one sense blinded, I learned there were some things I could control, and some things I could not, but I had a choice on where to concentrate my energies. Would they be positive or negative? The choice was mine, and if I wanted to live, they *had* to be positive.

We were given daily readings from the Bible and other sources. One of the suggested readings was called "Redeeming Love." It was a modern version of the story in the Book of Hosea concerning his relationship with the prostitute Gomar. The analogy was that a person with ED, and everyone else for that matter, makes mistakes. We repeatedly commit sins over and over, but God will always forgive us. But, if we keep making mistakes over and over where ED is concerned, there would be dire consequences in this life, even if God forgave us. Such a simple concept and it took me decades to understand it.

Despite the long drive from Las Vegas, Art visited me every weekend, and I can't put into words what it meant to me. Most of the time, he just sat there holding my hand, speechless. I never stopped asking him to validate what I was doing. Was it okay for me to be here? Was he getting along on his own? Of course, if he said yes, that meant I was worthless to him, so I needed him to tell me how much he missed me. He did.

That old habit was one of the hardest to break. I had never had an opinion of my own. I constantly strove to be an extension of Art's feelings and emotions. I still needed his approval for everything, even my therapy. Although they taught it to me at Remuda, I didn't truly understand, until I was away from Remuda, that Art's opinion wasn't the important thing. Mine was!

Some of my health problems were getting worse. The abdominal pain was nearly constant and the bowels remained balky. They were afraid I had a bowel obstruction, and I might be forced to leave. The thought chilled my heart with terror. I prayed, and God's answer this time was yes. He let it pass (so to speak) for now, so I could continue my journey.

In February, David and Kathy came to visit. It was wonderful and I enjoyed every moment of it. But, as they left, my fear about going home resurfaced. It was safe here. Life was structured, and help for any problem was readily at hand. For the first time in my life, I had completely relinquished control of my life to others. The thought of going home, and being in control of this new me was terrifying.

We were all working on our life story, and had to present it to Home Group. As I shared my life with them, the other women developed a new respect for me. I could see it in their faces.

Discovering the Monster Within

Two days later, one of the counselors told me that one of the girls, trusted me, and only me, and asked if I would be her safe person. A safe person, which each of us had, was a sounding board that you could bounce anything off of, and they would keep it in complete confidence. If you had a problem you weren't ready to share with staff, you could go to your safe person with it.

My joy at being the object of such a trust was shattered two days later when the same girl confronted me about how intimidating my love of God was and that my zeal was too much for her. Even my love for God was a problem. Would I ever learn to stop hurting people? Would I ever get it right? I prayed about it and the next day she came to me and told me everything was okay again. It was her problem, and not mine, and God had helped her understand that. Would He ever get it through my thick skull that everyone else's problems were not mine?

As I watched my comrades in arms battle the monster, I became acutely aware that their own feelings of self-worth was as bad or worse than mine, something I didn't think was possible. They formed little cliques where they criticized, lied and denied, deflecting the real issues away from themselves. Each of them subjugated her identity to the clique, and the clique became their personality. How sad they are, I said to myself, and a little voice whispered in my ear, "What about you, Patricia? Isn't that what you've been doing all your life, hiding behind your self-imposed wall of self-loathing? Have you ever had any emotions that were your own and not a reflection of someone else? This time, I knew it was not ED's voice I heard, but Someone who loved me despite myself.

Near the end of February, in a session with Rob, he unlocked one of the problems I couldn't solve. He helped me to see the connection between Art and my father. He told me that I had never grieved the fact that I didn't have a true father-daughter relationship with my father. I had never grieved for my lost childhood. When something is lost, a person must grieve that loss so life can go on. If the grief remains, the person is trapped in the unresolved emotion and it stunts their emotional growth. It leaves a deep, unfilled pit in one's emotional personality. It locks the child in a prison of blighted emotion.

"You have to grieve for what you cannot have, to make room for what you can have," he told me. "You never had a traditional father, and you never will have. Let that go and turn the space over to what you do have; a husband who loves you. If you don't believe that, consider the fact that he has stuck with you beyond the limits of reason. If there is something in your relationship that you want but can't have, grieve and let it go."

"Well, I do wish that Art was more romantic," I said with a sigh.

"If he doesn't have that characteristic, is it harmful to you? If it isn't, grieve and let it go. Grieve his lack of romance and celebrate his kindness to you. Don't hold onto and try to fix what you can't fix. Grieve and let it go," he added quietly.

How often I had done that. When Art was sad, or angry about something, I tried to fix it, when it was not in my power to do so. Instead of grieving the fact that it was beyond my control and rejoicing the fact that he shared his trouble with me, I kept trying to fix those troubles for Art. Finally, Rob had put it into perspective for me, and God had helped me understand it.

That's when I realized that Rob was right about what he calls, "the tapes in our head." Our minds function like a tape player. It carries the definition of 'self' imprinted on its surface, placed there by a lifetime of learning and experience. If the encoded information is incorrect and tells us that we are not worthy, we're wrong, we're inferior, we don't deserve to be happy, then we react like Pavlov's dogs responding appropriately to the lie as it is played for us during the stresses of life. Soon, I ignored the imperfections on the tapes and allowed myself to react to life's stresses with the destructive behaviors of anorexic and bulimic behavior.

It was time to erase that defective material and reprogram the tape. It wouldn't be easy, but I was determined to try. Not only did the tape have to be reprogrammed, my head had to believe the new data, and my heart had to embrace it.

A classic example is a simple compliment. It terrifies me and the panic nearly overwhelms me. The negative tape plays mocking commentary about the falseness of the compliment. I'm not worthy of praise. I don't deserve it. I deserve only derision. This person is making a fool of you. It's a joke. That's my Pavlovian response to the good-natured comment of a friend. I'm working on the new tape I so badly need.

As the days passed, I realized that many of the girls respected me because I never gave up. At my age, I had chosen to seek help rather than to die. My struggle was somehow inspirational to them. Instead of feeling good that I was helping them in some small way, I felt stupid, weak and sinful for waiting so long to seek help. The negative tape rolled, and the Pavlovian response kicked in. But, at least I can hear the scratches on the false tapes now.

Interestingly, my nursing skills tape is not flawed. That was one thing I did on my own. When I am in that element, I can fly. When the girls found out I was a nurse, they sought me out as the guru on life and health. I was careful not to become involved in the nursing care they were getting from staff. It was all first class and deserves only commendation. But simple hygiene questions, birth control issues and small things they wanted to know I readily supplied. I was humbled by their trust, and I gave them good advice. I think I benefited as much from the giving as they did from the receiving. It's in my genes. I was born to help others. God gave me that gift.

As March blew in like a Lion, whipping the desert sand into stinging brown clouds, we pointed towards family week. Each of us worked to polish our life story presentation and our letter of commitment. We continued to read parts aloud to each other in Home Group. It was always a very scary experience for me. I was baring my soul to a group of relative strangers. I'm still not sure how I was able to do it. Well, yes I do. God helped me.

"Family Nights" were fun. These were with our Remuda family, not our nuclear ones, and included everyone, not just Home Group. We popped popcorn, watched movies in our pajamas, worked puzzles and did girl talk. It was a slumber party all over again. I felt like a teenager, the teenager I had wanted to be, rather than the teenager circumstance forced me to be. It was a great stress reliever. In the relaxed atmosphere the conversation occasionally turned serious, and I discovered that many of them were more terrified than I was.

As each of us confronted our own visage of the monster, some of the girls got worse, and the overall tension became palpable. Two of the girls developed tremors so badly that they were confined to wheel chairs.

Fear spread as a brushfire does through the community. Was a virus attacking us? Were they faking? Would there be an epidemic? Unable to avoid being caught up in the moment, I wanted to imitate an ostrich and sick my head in the sand, or run away and hide. Panicky, I called Art. His calm reassurance saved me, again.

On the night before one of Art's visits, I was seized with the unreasonable fear that something bad had happened, or would happen, to him. ED was trying every thing that he could think of to take my concentration away from healing and thwart the progress I had made. ED thought a first class panic attack would work. It almost did, but not quite. When Art walked through the door, I felt as if I had just won the lottery.

Retrospectively, the source of my anxiety *was* that progress. Rob had gently rubbed the outer layer of scales from my eyes. All my life it had been me, me, me. I was the epicenter of everything. All that happened in my universe was either my fault or my responsibility. But, I had never taken responsibility for me. I was so busy trying to fix everything or make everybody else happy, that I never had time to make myself happy.

Rob helped me to look at my emotional self truthfully, and I began to realize that my data input was flawed, my processor broken and my storage device was off line. It was imperative that I once again focus on me, but with a new data set and new equipment. Putting aside Art, the family, and other girls at the ranch, I got the message and started the retooling process.

This was real progress, but it jacked up my anxiety. I began to feel like a machine. I still didn't have a 'me'. Was I doing what God wanted me to do? Why didn't I feel the emotions that the other girl's expressed? I went to my source of help in times of trouble and prayed to God for guidance.

It was a rare, raw, rainy day, in the desert when we had our body image challenge. As part of this exercise, we were given a piece of string and asked, without physically putting it around our waists, to make ourselves a belt. Mine wrapped around me more than twice. Despite my progress, I still saw a fat, acne scared woman I never was. It reinforced that what I had been seeing for forty years, and still saw, was a lie.

Next, we went to a clothing store, and while I was contemplating a dress, I tripped over a clothes rack and broke my toe! I just *love* osteoporosis. As I did with everything else, I put on my brave smile, minimized the discomfort and limped through the day.

The meals reinforced the fact that I was moving forward. After spending the rest of the morning trying on clothes, we went out to lunch. I ate pizza and salad! That evening at dinner, I had soup and half a sandwich. The lessons of the day and my successful encounter with food filled me with resolve to continue working to get well. ED, however, choked on the pizza.

Three days later, chapel was held on a mountainside where there were panoramic stations depicting the life and death of Jesus. I was so excited about the trip that even the light rain that began to fall couldn't dampen my spirits.

When we got there, it was much colder than I anticipated. Sleet and snow pelted down from a pewter sky. I wasn't dressed warmly enough, and I reacted as I always do to cold. My lips, nose, ears, toes, fingers, and any other protuberant part exposed to the elements turned blue.

Noticing my plight, Rob, in an act of kindness I shall never forget, took off his coat and made me put it on. Assuring me that he was used to the cold, he insisted that I wear it the rest of the afternoon.

I was humbled beyond belief. ED pushed play and the defective tape hissed, "Unworthy! Unworthy!" in my ear. When I flipped the switch to off, ED went postal. I didn't care. I was able to ignore him. Rob's act of kindness filled me with courage. Maybe, just maybe, if I was worth that much in Rob's eyes, how much more must I be worth to the man this mountain honored and to his Father who loved me fat or skinny. I doubled my resolve to stop desecrating His temple.

As I made final preparations for facing my family, I didn't want to hurt anyone, but I had to face the pain if I wanted to live. I love Art and I wanted to go home with him a better mate than I had been. That night, I wrote in my diary, "Am I a person? Do I feel? Will I ever be whole?" Unable to answer the question, I placed it all in the hands of God and prepared to meet my family. Ananias was coming to take the rest of the scales from my eyes.

Family week, near the end of therapy, is a major focus of the process. It is a time when you meet with your family in a loving confrontation about the damage ED has done to them, too. Carolyn's words, "I used to lay awake nights wondering whether or not you were going to die," rang in my ears.

Family Week is titled, Truth in Love, and that title tells the story of the week. The first is Truth. I was learning the truth about myself. While my whole life had been spent distorting how I pictured myself, I now had to look into the mirror and see the physical wreck I had really become. The same was true about what other people said to me, how I perceived what they said, and how I reacted to it. Now, I had to listen to what they were saying and really hear it, in front of witnesses! Those are daunting tasks if you live with ED.

As difficult as that was, accepting the truth about what ED had done to the members of my family was even harder. One-by-one, I went through my family and catalogued the damage I had done to them. When I finished, tears stained my cheeks.

The last truth, that cut the deepest, was the realization that although I blamed the monster for all the damage I had done, ED was my personal creation. ED was my child, my alter ego. In the laboratory of my mind, I had created a monster as deadly as any Dr. Frankenstein could conjure up in his mountain top castle. For four decades he ravaged the country-side of my life. Now, armed with torches and pitchforks supplied by the Burgomasters at Remuda, it was time to destroy the creature. Since the creature was a part of me, I wondered if I could survive the mob.

As for the rest of my family, my sisters knew I was there. My brother Dave was the only one I hadn't told I was going. It was up to me to decide who I would invite to family week. Art, the boys and their wives were on the guest list. With all my heart, I wanted Carolyn to come to be part of my healing and perhaps her own. God is about love, and forgiveness and second chances. I prayed that she had enough of God's love in her heart that she would help me take this important step. Since it was beyond my control, I placed it in God's hands, addressed her invitation and prayed she would come.

To supply the ammunition for the presentation, I wrote to each of my invited loved ones to tell me what damage my monster had done to them. I instituted the process by telling them what damage I felt I had caused them. Apologizing to them, I asked them to forgive me in my portion of the invitation.

David's wife, Kathy, chose not to come, because she had not been in my life very long at this point, and, it was extremely difficult for her to get off work for the time it would take to complete the program. I understand why she didn't come, but I wish she had. It would have provided her a unique insight into the dynamics of the family she had joined by marriage.

I kept the notes I used to write the letters to each of them. Calvin's is taped. It's taped because I ripped it up while filling it out. Determined to make it perfect and get every detail correct, I couldn't get it exactly the way I wanted it. Although I thought there were more forms, it was the last one I had, so I had to tape it together. It was a learning experi-ence.

We were required to hand in the forms to Rob. When he saw the tape, a smile crossed his lips as he immediately diagnosed my problem and helped me deal with it.

"Nobody's perfect, Pat," Rob told me. "God doesn't expect us to be perfect. He knows we're not. He knows we're flawed. You have to realize that, too. God expects you to *seek* perfection and do the best you can. You can't expect yourself to be perfect. None of us can be."

With that sound advice in mind, I finished my letters and sent them on their way.

My heart was on my sleeve as I awaited the responses. God answered my prayer, but this time, the answer was no.

Carolyn wasn't coming. She had married the man whose children she was originally hired to care for, and had done so without so much as a note to us. She did not want to leave her step-children. Tragically, even though she would be at Remuda, she said that she did not feel safe with me. I found that hard to accept. How could she be in danger in an institution in front of a live audience? Was she afraid of me, or was she afraid to face her own emotions?

Even harder was the salutation on the correspondence. "I love you," it said. They were merely words so easy to say at a distance. But, her action toward me, at a time when I needed love, if not mother-daughter love, at least Christian love, sent another message. Her behavior told me that she had neither in her heart for me.

Realizing how wounded I was, Rob wrote to her and asked her to come. He told her how important it was to my therapy, how much he believed it would help both of us, and how much I truly wanted her to come. His Christian concerns were answered with a callous rejection.

Unable to believe that a truly Christian daughter could feel this way about her mother, Rob called her on the phone. She was curt and abrasive to him. Accusing him of harassment, she demanded that he leave her alone.

"Don't ever try to contact me again," she snapped before hanging up.

Discovering the Monster Within

When he relayed the incident to me, Rob was flustered. "In all my years of counseling, no one has ever accused me of anything like that. Really, Pat, I wasn't harassing her, I was only trying to let her know how important this was to you and to encourage her to come. What's wrong with her, Pat?"

"Welcome to the club, Rob," I replied. "Now you know what I'm up against."

Carolyn also returned my letter of apology and request for forgiveness, unopened, inside another envelope. Rob found this behavior equally mystifying.

Carolyn requested no further contact from me, while I was at Remuda, but I kept the letter. On my last day at the ranch, I put it into another envelope, just as she had done to me, and mailed it back to her. I reasoned that this was an old contact, not a further one, so I could send it. That was the last contact I had with the daughter I love. As far as I am concerned, "the ball is in her court." I have done all I can do. It's up to God now.

To my letters to the family week invitees, the following is what I believe I had taken away from them by living with ED.

From Carolyn, I stole her childhood, although I don't know if she agrees or not. I placed her on a pedestal and tried, in my defective way, to relive my own lost childhood through her. I was as bad as the athlete-want-to-be berating the little leaguer because he or she made and error, or fighting with another parent over a hockey game. That never works, and it cost me my little girl. If you ever read this, Carolyn, I am truly sorry.

I took from David the time and patience to recognize his individuality. His hyperactivity was a significant enough problem. My perfectionism and mood swings crated an unstable environment that made it impossible for him to have even the semblance of a normal childhood.

My temper fed Calvin's innate obstinacy and created the milieu for his rebellion. Most rebellious children are telling their parents that they want attention and love. They want the lines to be drawn. It tells them they're loved. I think it was that way with Cal, too. But he couldn't get that kind of satisfaction from our attempts to draw those lines, because he was afraid his mother was going to die.

Art, what can I say about Art. I stole from him the wife he married and traded her in for a starving, withered shrew he never signed on for. The communication, understanding and marital support so necessary in a healthy relationship, vanished under ED's corrosive influence.

I stole a loving, giving companion and the sexual partner (the way my body looks, not my desire or our activity,) that he deserved. I took years of peace and growth and in its place instilled a fear into him that created a confused, closed-up, lonely man. There were other slights, but perhaps the way I verbally abused him in front of our friends and neighbors was heart wrenching. The pain and grief I felt writing those confessions is still impossible for me to translate into words.

My invitees wrote back to me with the changes they had seen in me, thanks to ED. For the children, this was a relative question, since none of them could remember me without it. Their older brother ED was in the family long before any of them were.

The most significant thing all of them noticed was the obvious physical deterioration.

"It's heart-rending to see her body so emaciated."

"We don't understand how she can function when her body is so abused."

"It's difficult to make any other observations because she's been that way most of her life."

"Our biggest fear is that if she were to become seriously ill or injured, like in a car accident, her body wouldn't be able to handle the stress of that kind of injury."

"When we were children, we were always afraid she might die."

"She is emotionally erratic and inconsistent. She can focus on negative comments and puts herself on the defensive when no intentional "attack" was made. Then, she acts out by closing in on herself and not eating. This kind of thinking is as harmful as the physical aspects of her disease."

Despite my apprehension, it was wonderful to see everyone as they arrived on Sunday. Filled with my new insight, it was exciting, intimidating and humiliating to consider opening myself up, to make myself vulnerable. Could I finally admit my pain and illness and ask for help and forgiveness in front of all those people? The hard work I had done with the Remuda professionals was about to be severely tested.

I didn't enter the week alone. I got so many prayers and words of encouragement that it made me feel foolish that I had never asked for help before. Each day began at the chapel service, and the closeness to God helped calm me for the task. I would never be alone as long as I lived. God was with me.

When the families were settled in the guest quarters, the sessions opened with a welcoming speech. They were given a thumbnail sketch of what we had experienced at the ranch. Then, the families went off to classes with the staff and without us. Staff discussed the recovery process, symptoms of backsliding and what to say and not to say to the recovering patient with the families.

On the second day, we began classes together in problem resolution and communication. During this time, we ate separately from our families. Days three to five involved our presentations. My presentation was on day four, and I felt grateful that I was able to see the other presentations before my turn came. At least I knew what was expected of me.

The classes we took together were emotionally charged and filled with energy. One of the important lessons concerned family dynamics and the methods ED used to infiltrate families. We learned that it begins subtly, as it did in my case. Slowly, my behavior drove a wedge between Art and me, warped my children's view of life and cost me my daughter.

Another class involved communication skills and the flaws that were in them. Each class used worksheets that Art and I filled out separately. Then, we discussed the sheets and the things we had written on them.

It was apparent that our communication problems involved only two things, listening and hearing.

Often, I didn't listen. It was more important for self-centered me to form my next point than listen to what the presenter was telling me. When I did hear, I didn't hear what was really said. I could take the most innocent phrase or comment and wrap it into a criticism or self-condemnation. As ED progressed and my alcohol consumption escalated, my tongue became a lethal weapon. I had unwittingly become the reincarnation of my father. With flawed input and faulty processing, the output resembled computer-speak. It was "gigo," garbage in, garbage out.

A class on making choices of how we hear or interpret followed that class. See, God always sends us what we need, even if we think we don't want it. The important lesson was still that everything wasn't about me. I could actually choose to listen to what Art was saying, rather than thinking about how what he was saying related to me. Not only listen, but hear and understand how much of what he said to me was filled with love for me. How I wish I had learned that forty years ago.

Taking over our power, forging growth, God's place in our marriage and family, respecting individuality and an individual's special abilities and talents, and last but not least loving ourselves were other topics we explored together in this whirlwind week. With the help of the Remuda staff, I was able to attack each of the areas with new weapons and a new mind set aimed at healing rather than just interaction. Without that understanding, simply talking about the problems is not enough. Running the gamut of emotions through humility, shame, remorse and joy, I negotiated the week in a cloud of emotions.

We learned together, laughed together, loved together, cried together, forgave and asked for forgiveness. Most importantly, God was there with us, as the conductor of a human orchestra gradually turning a sad sonata into a symphony of triumph.

My big day finally arrived. Filled with trepidation, I pursued my morning ablutions in a spirit of prayer even before I went to chapel. I would need all the help I could get. Susan and Liz, two of my Home Group sisters, paved the way on day three, and we witnessed the remarkably emotional scenes as they interacted with their families. I felt confident and ready.

The first part of the presentation involved my life story from my childhood to the doors of Remuda. I emphasized my feelings of low self-esteem, inferiority, my shame at being a girl, my shame at what had happened to me, and shame at my addictive personality that included cleanliness, perfectionism, victimization and compulsiveness. They are addictions as surly as the habituation to alcohol I had developed! Art later told me that this portion of my presentation was filled with deep remorse for what I had done. I'm glad it came across that way. That's how I felt.

Addressing the members of my family, I apologized to each of them individually and asked them to forgive me. As I did, they responded to me verbally. Each of them accepted my apology, forgave me, and asked me to forgive them for what they had done to enable ED to live with us so long. A tidal wave of love washed over me creating such warmth and peace that I felt as if God had enclosed the entire family in a huge, bright bubble of His grace!

After all the pain I had caused them, to receive such love from the dearest people in my life nearly broke my heart. David, who is so much like me that he seldom shows any emotion was a sobbing mass of Jell-O when he responded to me.

As tears tracked down his cheeks he said to me, "You are the most important person in my life." When we embraced, I couldn't speak, because I was sobbing just as hard as the power of forgiving love engulfed us both. The tears of my oldest son on my cheek were a healing balm that soothed my soul like nothing else could.

Calvin, my emotional one, had no trouble forgiving me and thanked me for helping him grow up. I'm sure he wasn't thanking me for the old fashioned donnybrooks of his childhood but helping him truly grow up. We have developed closeness just from Cal being Cal. His tears, filled with love, forgiveness and God's grace were sweet. Both my sons covered me with compassion, respect and admiration.

Then it was my loving, insightful daughter-in-law Tina's turn, and if Tina has never hugged you, you have never been hugged. When my gorgeous Tina wraps her arms around you, you can literally feel the God driven love radiating from her.

By the time I got to the love of my life, I was a basket case. Art was by far the most compassionate and loving. His tears washed away forty years of pain. Art told me I was his life and without me, he had no life at all. When we got up to embrace each other the entire room was awash with our love for each other, and God's love for all of us.

Among so many other crushing emotions, I felt their respect. After all I had done to them; they still loved and respected me. God is good, and He blessed the Burkley family that day in Arizona.

The family's emotional roller coaster still wasn't at the station; there was one more hill to negotiate. On the last day of family week, another young woman faced the music, and she was completely alone. None of her family could be with her. She is a wonderful girl, with a gentle, loving spirit, brightness and without guile. So naïve that she is hard to believe, we identified with her need.

Since everyone must present to someone, Sarah inquired if she could present to us. We agreed, and she asked Art to be her father and Tina to be her mother. They acted out what she went through, and just hearing her outlandish tale and realizing she had no support at all broke our hearts. So unsophisticated and vulnerable, she needed a family, and we became hers for a day.

To say, "God works in mysterious ways," is to repeat an overused cliché. But, He did that day for both Sarah and the Burkley family. Since I've left Remuda, Art and I have taken a personal and active interest in Sarah's life. We have chosen to become a loving support system for her, as she attends college, and she has replaced for us some of the pain we suffered in losing our own daughter.

Discovering the Monster Within

The last assignment of family week was an after letter from the family answering two simple questions, with very complex answers. What changes have you noticed in me? And, any concerns or fears related to my leaving treatment and coming back home?

Their response to the first question was nearly unanimous. "You are calmer than when you entered therapy and more at peace with yourself. You're listening more and not taking offense at every little thing anyone says to you. Your positive exuberance is still there, but now it seems tempered. You're not afraid to just sit and be "Pat." We have never seen you so ready for help and are encouraged by the range of foods you will now eat."

All my men had the same concern, my relapse. No question that would be important. My sons independently commented on my drive to do what I set out to do and prayed it would be enough to prevent any backsliding.

Art had a separate fear. He was concerned about putting pressure on me. He also realized what I needed was love and acceptance for who I was, not what I was, or what I did or looked like. I would need his help on that score, since I had just learned to accept those things about myself. Art's next statement filled me with gratitude.

"You have now, and probably always have had, an inner strength of both faith and personal values beyond anyone I've ever met."

But, it was Tina who expressed my own fears in her insightful response.

"The concern I have is that after so many years, it'll be too easy to slip into the same old routine; mostly that it'll be easier to limit your menu so it gets smaller and smaller instead of expanding it to a broader range of foods. Since you're a nurse, and a logical, intelligent person, I'm afraid you'll rationalize your behavior into eating only the things with the best nourishment. You relied heavily on supplements to fill in the needs once she realized your body was betraying you, (protein supplements, calcium supplements and the like.) I'm afraid this logic and rationalization will take you back to the behavior."

The House of Judah

The concerns she enumerated were on my mind. But, I had others as well. Here, things were safe, structured, and at the slightest setback, there was someone to hold my hand, to give me advice, to set me back on the right path, to ignore my excuses. Once I left the womb of Remuda, and cut the cord with my therapists there, I was on my own. Did I have what it takes? Would I be strong enough? I felt I was, but only God knew for sure, so I placed everything in His capable hands and continue to ask Him for daily counsel and assistance.

Friday night and Saturday were family pass times. I went to dinner with the family and later, we just wandered the small town of Wickenburg. It was wonderful to be away with family.

On Saturday we went to a renaissance fair near Apache Junction, Arizona with my family. We met Kathy and her parents there and had a wonderful day. Tina and I even rode an elephant! I couldn't ride horses as Remuda, but I could ride elephants at the fair.

When the family said good-by on Sunday, I was so full of joy and peace that I couldn't feel sad that they were leaving. Besides, I knew that in another week I would be home with Art again, for good. He had written to me every day and visiting every allowed weekend while I was at the ranch. I couldn't wait to get home to him.

My last week at Remuda was spent reviewing signs of backsliding, where to find support groups and medical help. There was a gradual adjustment from the highly structured living conditions of the past two months to a more relaxed atmosphere in anticipation of returning to the real world where I would have to put into practice what I had learned. *That* was a scary thought.

A new staff member came on board that week. She arranged an outing for three of us. The other two women chose not to go because we were not going to go to the movies. I felt they didn't go because I was going. At the first challenge, it was back to me …me…me. When I realized it was their problem, not mine, I felt better. But, it foreshadowed the struggles to come.

Discovering the Monster Within

So, off we went, the two of us, in a fifteen-passenger van belonging to the ranch. Yakking away, and unfamiliar with the highway, she turned down a dirt road, which was not a road at all. It was a desert wash, and we sank up to our hubcaps in mire. Here we were, out in the boonies, miles from nowhere, and hopelessly stuck. After an hour of trying everything we could think of, we were still stuck. I called God's AAA service on my prayer radio.

A truck appeared and our spirits were buoyed until we saw the passengers. Two scraggly, hippy-looking men were inside. When they stopped, thoughts of rape and pillage flashed through my head. Instead of Attila the Hun, they turned out to be Mother Theresa clones. They were absolutely two of the most likeable men you'd ever want to meet. Be careful, "lest you meet angels unaware."

Literally everyone in the desert drives a pickup, and a second one loomed on the horizon. This time, it was a family with two small children. They stopped, too. Why wouldn't they? They were stereotype Middle America, and we were damsels in distress. The father joined our two new friends in the mire.

I thought a man drove the third truck, until the driver got out of the cab. An elderly woman was in the passenger seat, and the woman driver was complete with sleeveless T-shirt and tattoos. She proved to be as kind and thoughtful as her appearance was hard. While helping to disgorge our vehicle, she found a heart-shaped stone and presented it to me. It remains among my treasures.

Getting the heavy vehicle out was a chore. They did everything imaginable including, blocks and wedges, letting air out of the tires and a dozen other things. Their labor was finally rewarded with a resounding "smuck" as the van released to solid ground. Spurning our offers of reward, this wonderful band of Samaritans smiled, shook our hands, hugged us, wished us well, and went on their way. I think they were real people, but they certainly acted like angels.

This experience was a dab of cement on my building project with God. I always knew God was there. Didn't He save me in a snowstorm?

Didn't He get me home with the sun in my face when I was virtually blind? Of course He did! Sending two women stranded in the desert a trio of vehicles filled with wise men, and women, to solve their problem was just one more proof of life for God. He is alive.

Not only is He alive, He is always teaching. That night, He taught me that no matter how helpless the situation appears on the surface, there is a way out, and no matter how someone looks, it's how they act that counts. Thanks God, for the reminders.

Back on solid ground with hunger gnawing at our bodies, we went to find food. I ordered a pasta dish and was able to eat a significant part of it. Afterwards, we went to a Dairy Queen, owned by the driver's father. While he checked the van for significant damage, we hung out at the ice cream parlor.

While we were there, an entire bus load of teenagers came by following a basketball game. It was great to vicariously share their enthusiasm. When her father gave the van a clean bill of health, we headed for Remuda after a memorable night on the town. All the way home, we giggled like teenagers on the way to the prom.

Awaking on the last day at Remuda Ranch, I asked God for peace, wisdom and health. It was scary. I didn't want to hurt anyone, and I needed to reassure the other girls that I was no more special in God's eyes than they were. It was important for me to feel peace in their hearts and mine as we parted.

There was also anger and sadness for ED who had damaged so many wonderful women. Each time someone leaves, they are honored and prayed for at their last meal. I knew it was going to happen and the positive strokes made me feel uneasy, but less so than I thought they would. Thank you God.

I also wondered if I would go back to Art healed enough. It was an emotional day filled with hugs and tears and laughter. Shortly before Art arrived to pick me up, one of the more touching moments of that last day occurred.

Discovering the Monster Within

As I went through the morning, I found myself trying to close off my emotions, since I felt so close to so many of the girls. They knew the real me and accepted me as is. That was a very important step in my growth. Then, one special woman stepped forward and told me that she couldn't have made it without me. I spent a great deal of time with her that day. I asked her to help me pack so I could have more time with her. It was a wonderful experience for both of us, and another lesson from God. Live your life for good every day. You never know when you are going to be an example. Try to be a good one.

Though it was difficult to leave Remuda, I was so anxious to be with Art, and feel him close to me, that I wanted to leave. I was certain that all was well and in complete denial that I would ever let the monster in again. Little did I anticipate the struggles that lay ahead as deep inside ED pouted and bided his time.

I was reluctant to go straight home and back to the old routine too quickly. I wanted time with Art to share, relax and talk over what had happened to us, about our future, and the help I would need from him. He agreed.

As we drove away from the ranch, I felt relief, fear, peace, terror and anticipation all rolled into one. Most of all, I was thankful for the Heavenly Father and all His blessings. We drove to Phoenix, and I remember eating sherbet and two cups of yogurt, something I wouldn't consider prior to Remuda.

Two days later, we went to Sabino Canyon in the Catalina Mountains, and after a great day and restful night, when I slept better than I had in months, we drove to Mt. Lemon near Tucson and met David. That night, he grilled seafood and made noodles which I was able to eat without difficulty. After a visit to Prescott, we headed home.

My joy at being home is still indescribable. It was both good and scary to be there, but I was there and determined that I would do everything in my power to keep ED outside in the blazing Las Vegas sun. But, I knew I could do it, with the help of the same God that took the scales from Paul's eyes, and mine.

CHAPTER 14

Call 911

The physical toll that ED imparts upon his victims is as brutal as its emotional effects, and the body I took with me to Remuda was in shambles. Though I have mentioned some of them in passing, I think it is imperative that I enumerate them. This affords a proper perspective on the physical deterioration resulting from slow, sustained, deliberate starvation.

Young anorexics stand a twelve times greater chance of dying than age matched controls. Cardiac arrest or suicides top the list of causes, but complications of substance abuse and severe psychiatric illness are not far behind. Anorexic's die at the rate of five percent per decade increasing to twenty percent if the disease lasts over twenty years. At two times twenty I shudder to think of what my potential mortality was. This isn't a fad diet; it's a fatal disease.

I find myself wondering why none of the doctors or dentists I saw over the years ever mentioned anorexia to me. To be honest, some anorexics may be severely ill and have a normal physical exam and normal lab studies. Some of us feel ill. Others, like me, feel deceptively healthy. Perhaps some of the doctors did mention my weight along the way, but I didn't hear them if they did. I'm sure many of them wrote the diagnosis on the chart but never discussed it with me. I wouldn't have listened if they had.

Starvation is a disease that affects the entire organism. Anorexics feel dull, listless, depressed, and have trouble thinking or concentrating as the central nervous system is robbed of vital nutrition. The heart related symptoms include slow irregular pulse, dizziness and low blood pressure, shortness of breath and chest pains, feeling constantly cold with blue lips and fingers, and unfortunately sudden death. Bones demineralization occurs and bones fracture with a seven times greater incidence, including stress fractures without significant trauma.

Purging leads to enamel erosion, cavities and gum disease, a sign called, "Chipmunk Cheeks" from swollen salivary glands due to vomiting and a constant sore throat, pain in the esophagus simulating cardiac pain, bloody vomit from small esophageal rips, esophageal rupture, gastric retention, gastric rupture after a big purge, and severe electrolyte imbalance that can lead to cardiac arrest. Constipation is a constant companion of the anorexic.

Laxative abuse adds bleeding, bloating, dependency, electrolyte imbalance and dehydration. Pretty picture, isn't it?

The summary of my pregnancies sounds like an ob/gyn textbook. Two miscarriages and a baby born so prematurely that he could not survive is more than coincidence. Both my boys tried to deliver early, and in the only term pregnancy I had with Carolyn, was complicated by troublesome bleeding. Every one of the children was well below the average birth weight. I believe that even though I tried to protect my little passengers with a diet I thought was good for them, the vehicle in which they were riding was a dangerous place for them to be. I have to conclude that the problems I had with childbearing were related to ED.

I can't find data to prove it, but I believe that when the body is in such negative nutritional balance, it cannot stand the extra strain of carrying a fetus. My disease was less severe when Carolyn was born. Was that why I had less trouble with her? Since ED stops the periods of many Anorexics, interferes with fertility, and destroys relationships to the point that pregnancy is not an issue, this may be hard data to accumulate. Still, I think it would be worthwhile to try.

Bulimic behavior does a number on the teeth. By age twenty-five, the corrosive effects of the hydrochloric stomach acid that daily bathed my teeth during purging removed all the enamel from my teeth that were not genetically strong in the first place. I began a long series of caps, root canals, dentures, and implants. I am still plagued with recurrent gum problems due to my impaired resistance to gingival bacteria. I remember taking the children to the dentist with me in their car beds due to the long dental procedures. No dentist ever asked me about bulimic behavior.

As physicians searched for ways to reverse the catabolism that my eating behavior set in motion, they even gave me medicine for low thyroid function. Interestingly, if the thyroid function is truly low, one slows down, gets sluggish and gains weight. My hyperactive behavior certainly didn't fit the diagnosis. Still I was on thyroid medication for a year.

I have had any number of episodes of esophageal spasm that led to trips to the emergency department. I had every gastric test and examination know to mankind. They all turned up negative. How many of those were stress induced, psychosomatic, or ways to have attention drawn to myself? I have no idea. All of these things are part of ED's wardrobe. When I had these attacks, I couldn't eat anything for fear of the terrible discomfort the spasms caused, and ED was ecstatic about that.

After a period of chronic laxative abuse, the bowel's normal peristaltic activity that propels waste material through the large and small bowel slows down and then stops. The medical term for this phenomenon is paralytic ileus. My bowel quit working on a number of occasions. Most of the time, a nasogastric tube and suction drainage did the trick, and I could go home. Other times, I required hospitalization until the ileus resolved. Did I ever get scolded about my laxative use? No, most of the time, they didn't ask. On the rare occasion when they did, I lied about my actual consumption of cathartics.

Discovering the Monster Within

Three times in my life, I have had thrush, as a result of malnutrition. Thrush is an overgrowth of bacteria in the throat that produces pain and inflammation.

After being treated for the ulcer I developed after David was born, I enjoyed a period of relative health, free from any physical symptoms. That gave ED the opportunity to convince me that I was fine and everybody else was wrong. My system was somehow different. I didn't need what most others required for good health! So, I continued to live the lie.

With the combination of all these symptoms, my underlying problem should have been obvious to most of my treating physicians. Perhaps it was. Yet, none of them put pressure on me to seek counseling, see a psychiatrist or nutritional expert. I'm not sure if they didn't recognize the problem or if it was simpler to treat the physical symptoms and ignore the ED. Maybe less attention was paid to eating disorders then. I'm not sure. If I had been ready for help or could have been convinced to seek help, how different my life might have been.

By the time symptoms reappeared, I had far advanced disease. When I fell on New Year's Eve and fractured my elbow, ED alone wasn't to blame. More than one klutzy adult has broken a bone on a sheet of unseen ice. But, the fracture was treated and my calcium levels were never measured or commented upon. They already had to be dangerously low.

About that same time, my skin began to bruise and tear with the regularity of a ninety-year-old woman. Working at the psychiatric hospital was particularly hazardous to my health. For starters, I had innumerable injuries related to thin skin and malnutrition occurred. When the entire fat pad is gone under the skin, and the skin is stretched across bone like the head on a snare drum, it tears very easily.

We had old-fashioned beds there with manual cranks for raising the head of the bed. They folded back into the bed frame when not in use. Someone left a crank out, and making rounds on the nightshift in the dark, I bumped my shin on the crank handle. There is precious little padding over the shinbone in the healthy adult. In my case, there was none. The ensuing laceration necessitated an emergency department visit and stitches. My souvenir of the occasion is the scar on my leg.

Once while working with a violent patient, another significant injury occurred. She cornered me and kicked my legs, while two other women attempted to subdue her. Both my legs were ripped to shreds, but staffing was so bad that my supervisor doused me with peroxide and Neosporin, bandaged my legs and I continued my shift in the bloody pants.

Arriving home, I soaked the pants in cold water and fell into bed, planning an emergency department visit as soon as I had the strength to manage the trip. I fell asleep, and Carolyn found the pants. The poor child was frantic until she saw me and knew that I was okay. I drove myself to the hospital where they took pictures, and changed my dressings. My legs eventually healed with lots of scar tissue.

It seems as though my legs had a bull's eye painted on them. We usually passed out juice with the medications. While opening one of the industrial sized cans, I dropped it. It hit my leg and lacerated it again. By then I was on a first name basis with the suture tech at the emergency department. Yes, I am accident prone, and no my legs will never make Hollywood.

The most frightening time occurred during a scuffle when a patient slammed me up against the wall with his hands around my throat. In an attempt to rescue me, someone's arm twisted mine, and the skin on my forearm ripped. No sutures were required this time, but the trauma would never have affected a normal person.

I also had my first stress fracture of my foot while working there. I was fitted with a boot that I wore for about four weeks. A calcium substitute became a part of my diet from that point on. No bone density was done. The orthopedic surgeon said it wasn't necessary. He could see on the routine x-rays that I had osteoporosis, and a test to prove it would be a waste of money.

Achilles had his heel, and I have my legs. In 1992, I wrestled with the volcano in Hawaii and lost. I fainted from lack of energy, fell and lacerated my leg requiring thirteen stitches. That one took forever to heal.

By then, I thought my legs were so full of scar tissue they would be impervious to further trauma. Not so. In 1998, I injured my leg while moving a box and was later struck by a flying box propelled by the wind. The hematoma was so huge that it increased in size, spontaneously drained and produced a necrotic muscle bed that refused to heal. After literally hundreds of dressing changes and electrotherapy, it finally healed. These traumas, though significant, were not severe enough to produce these kinds of complications in a well-nourished individual. Thanks to my companion, ED, I was a walking complication, pun intended.

Every doctor I saw ran another battery of tests and came up with a couple of abnormal ones. That's the problem with doing a lot of medical tests. If one of them is out of whack, it requires a dozen more to prove you have nothing to be concerned about. In my case my ANA, anti-nuclear antibodies, levels were very high. When something attacks the nucleus of a healthy cell, the body forms antibodies against the attacker. These antibodies can be measured. A high level suggests that cells in the body are being attacked in great numbers, and that is usually cancer at work.

I was also making great big cells. Normal blood contains an occasional cell called macrocytes, because of their large size. Mine were even bigger than normal, and in the face of low protein levels, (if you don't eat protein, you have low levels) there could be a serious underlying problem. The result was three years with a cancer specialist. I saw him every six months and had a quart of blood drawn for all the tests. When the test results came back, I still didn't have a diagnosis.

In 1999, my leg gradually became red, swollen and extremely painful resulting in my trip to the Mayo Clinic in Scottsdale and the diagnosis of all my stress fractures. At least the casts were cool. I had three, one purple, one hot pink and one green. That place has panache.

The doctors there also found irregularities in my liver function. According to the specialist, the combination of malnutrition and alcohol consumption coupled with the liver problem was the cause of the macrocytosis. ED strikes again.

Over the past few years, I have been treated extensively for the osteoporosis. Oral medication as well as two, four-hour infusions of calcium have been used. With all that, I am barely holding my own in the calcium department.

Also, I had problems with a roller coaster heart beat. My pulse fluctuated between 48 and 170-180! When the heart raced, I got short of breath and had chest pain. The arteries in the heart passed muster, and I was medicated with a variety of medications and combinations of medication that did nothing. Eventually, in February 2002, they did an ablation of the electrical system of the heart to slow things down. I was on the table for four hours and had to lay flat for eight hours until they were able to stop the bleeding in the groin area. Lots of "normal" people have these kinds of problems with their heart, but it seemed a significant number of the women at Remuda had pulse problems of one sort or another.

I also kept having pain over the liver area that was pretty nasty at times. I had about every test imaginable, upper GI, gallbladder, CAT scan. You name it I had it done. They even did this wonderful new test to see if my gallbladder was obstructed. The resultant spasm of the gallbladder produced the equivalent of an acute gallbladder attack. Boy was that fun! Nothing was found, and no one asked me about laxative use.

While they tried to track the source of the abdominal pain down, I detached my retina. The black spot I noticed as the initial symptom remains. The brain is a wonderful and powerful machine, and it has trained itself to ignore the spot most of the time, except when I get tired. The more tired I am, the more likely I am to notice my little blind spot.

Was it ED or bad luck? Who knows? I believe that physicians get so busy trying to keep us alive, and avoid malpractice suits, that they don't have the luxury to check into our ancillary health problems. Although my eating disorder was certainly not ancillary, I think I understand why they didn't. Most physicians simply are not trained to handle eating disorders. There is a real need for physicians with that kind of compassion and expertise.

Recently, a dermatologist told me that my skin, and even my hair, showed the effects of malnutrition. Although the diagnosis was tongue twisting, it sounds worse than it really is. If thin skin and damaged hair follicles were the worse things I had to deal with, I'd be a happy camper.

My bladder has also become extremely thin and the muscle wall has lost its tone. This is called neurogenic bladder disease. It happens to lots of middle-aged women and the treatment is life-long medication. Although many women who do not have ED have this problem, I have been told that the severe nutritional depletion of a lifetime is partly to blame for my condition.

To illustrate the fragility of my body, in September of 2000, we had joined a health club. As I was reaching to pull down on a handle of one of the machines, I got a sharp pain in the middle of my chest. I fractured my sternum! Rest and if it hurts to do that, don't do that, was my prescription.

Although it occurred after we returned from Remuda, my most frightening health problem struck me on October 18, 2002. We went to Red Lobster for lunch, and abdominal pain began soon after. I tried to have a bowel movement to relieve the pain. I had been having some bowel problems and was on two stool softeners a day. These pains were like the ones the doctors had been previously unable to diagnose. As I walked down the hall in my home, it felt as if a Ninja assassin had stuck his short sword into my abdomen. Collapsing to the floor, I rolled on my side and tried to get up, but the pain was so awful I could only cry out for help. Art was in his garage workshop with the saw running and couldn't here me. After what seemed like an eternity, but was in reality only a few minutes, he heard my screams and came running.

We must have lots of emergencies in Las Vegas, because when Art called 911 he got put on hold . . . twice! When you are laying in the fetal position wracked by the most excruciating pain imaginable, it takes a long time for the ambulance to arrive. Trying to keep a brave front, I calmly explained to the ambulance attendants that I thought I had a bowel obstruction or perhaps a kidney stone, but that I was afraid I might have an aneurysm. They were amazed at my knowledge and my calm. It was all a sham. As soon as the words were out of my mouth, I surrendered to the fear and the pain.

They transported me to the hospital and for the next thirty-five hours tried to get me to drink CAT scan dye. The result was my imitation of a breeching sperm whale when I spewed the liquid back out. Finally, with no other choice, the doctor took me to surgery. On my way to the operating room, I prayed like I had not prayed in a long time.

My gut was completely obstructed, and I had perforated my stomach with associated peritonitis. According to the doctor, I was one sick cookie, but I didn't need him to tell me that. He had to resect a significant portion of damaged bowl that was tissue paper thin from years of chronic laxative abuse. Unsure if it would heal, he sewed me back together.

The next two days, I *knew* I was in trouble. I talked with God a lot, and told Him that I wasn't ready to come home yet, but told him I would trust Him, and His will be done. Thank God He heard me, and I healed up. But, it was a long slow process.

Once again, I owed my life to God and Remuda Ranch. Had this crisis occurred before I had gone there there, I don't believe I would have been strong enough to survive it. I certainly wasn't the picture of health, but I was stronger and better nourished than I was before I went to Remuda. The body needs fuel to mend, and although I was still on low octane, it was better than the nothing I was eating before.

Most of all, I felt bad for Art. Once again the ravages of ED had intruded on his life and left him playing nursemaid to a sickly mate.

Before I was released I had a follow up CAT scan, and they spotted an unusual shadow on my bones. Much deliberation later, they decided it was a benign thing called a bone island. For a while, the specter of cancer in my bones was with me, and I didn't like it. I had decided to live after trying to starve myself to death for forty years. I didn't want another setback.

For years, like many people, I suffered from a chronic infection of my great toenails. Gradually things got worse and the toes became sore and secondarily infected. The oral medicine used to treat these infections has a side effect of diarrhea, which I could ill afford, and some immune suppression so it was out of the question for me. So, off came the toenails! With prolonged soaking, Silvadene topically and antibiotic for the infection, the problem finally resolved.

That wasn't the only problem with my feet. Chronic loss of fat in the pads over the bones in my feet results in another source of chronic discomfort.

Quite an impressive list, isn't it? And, it doesn't include another sternum fracture in two thousand three, and a fractured foot and toes in two thousand four. Is the list as long as it's going to get? I doubt it. Have I damaged my body to the point where parts of it will continue to fail me? That's likely. What can I do about it? I can try to give my body the sound nutrition it needs, get the rest I need and pray that The Great Physician will continue to touch me with His healing hand.

CHAPTER 15

Road to Recovery Potholes and All

I t's been three short years since Remuda. If I were to tell you that I had this horrendous problem and my lifestyle of four decades completely under control after a couple of months at a girl's ranch in the desert, you would doubt my veracity, my sanity, or both and with good reason.

It has been over two years since I have indulged in any binge purge behavior, the longest since I can't remember when. I still must constantly battle the urge to restrict, but I am getting better at that. Still, when the stress levels get too high, it remains a safety valve for me, and I'm working on developing more healthy ones.

I am *not* cured, but I am recovering. "My name is Pat, and I have an Eating Disorder. I've not used laxatives in three years, nor binged, or purged in two years!" has become my battle cry. It's that kind of day-to-day struggle, but each day I'm getting stronger, and I struggle less.

When I left Remuda, I was filled with the confidence, peace and joy shared by many of those who have been there. I was filled with resolve. Never would I backslide into the sticky morass from which I had escaped. I was born again with the faith of Remuda, and with God's help it couldn't happen to me. After decades of damage to my family, my health and my friends, I was ready for a new life. My treatment team was lined up. The best friend and soul mate anyone could ever have was in the car with me, and, I was surrounded by God's love! What more did I need?

Back home, I met with my nutritionist first. Joanie knew that numbers ruled my life, and healthy eating was the important thing she tried to teach me. They told me at Remuda that I should weigh about one hundred ten pounds, but not a lot more because of the fragility of my bones; still, no scales for me. Joanie would handle that.

Besides nutrition, this wonderful woman also helped me realize that I needed to discover personal joy and something special for myself everyday. Not the old "myself" center of the universe; she who must spin the earth or it won't turn, but for the little girl trapped inside of me yearning to be free. She told me too many women are so busy giving, giving, giving, that they never take any time for themselves. That's me. My most important lesson was to learn that it was my responsibility to take time for myself. No one else could do it for me. It was time to stop trying to fix other's lives and fix my own.

Joanie taught me that by caring for myself, I was honoring God and my loved ones as well as myself. What an important step that was for me to take. It was a baby step at restoring a low self-esteem I carried with me as if it were an extra purse.

A major obstacle I must continually face is my obsessive behavior. Food labels are a classic example. The FDA's intent with the labels was to improve the nutrition of the nation, with special attention to the large number of overweight citizens among us. Detailed information concerning the calories and ingredients of every packaged food product in America is readily available on the wrapper or can. Even when there is nothing nutritional at all, as in diet soda, it still has to print a zero for everything.

I use them to the opposite extreme, as do most of us with ED. The folks at Remuda warned us against constantly searching for no fat, low fat, everything. I admit I have not yet broken that ritual, but I'm far better at it now that I was three years ago. If I have a choice between brand A's five grams of fat and brand B's six, brand A used to win every time. Now, it's not every time. God, and Art are gradually helping me change.

I still have problems with menus. It's not so much the menus as it is the decision of what I want, what's good for me, and what Art enjoys. Unfortunately, I find myself steering toward the shore of "safe" foods from the old days, such as salads with no dressing. Despite the daily challenge, I am inching my way toward a more normal daily fare.

The compulsion complicated my attempts to follow the food plan they outlined for me at Remuda. At first, I couldn't do it. I would obsess all day long about the menu, feeding Art and me with food that was appropriate for each of us rather than food for *both* of us. Starting with salads, egg whites, fresh fruit and vegetables, I continued to avoid the starches and desserts of my childhood. For years I would rather die than gain a gram of weight. Now, that drop dead weight is much higher but still not unlimited, thanks to bones with the tensile strength of spider webs.

My obsession carries over to clothes as well. What should I wear? Does my underwear match my outfit? I frequently bought inexpensive things and constantly reminded others how little they cost so they would know I wasn't indulging myself. How foolish. I'm still not extravagant, and never will be, but I don't do that anymore.

Joanie, shared with me that she matches underwear to outfit too. Instead of being ashamed of my compulsion, she said that everyone is different, and I should embrace that quality and use it for the good things it can do and not beat myself up with it. "Celebrate your differences and make them positives rather than negatives," she told me. It was sound advice and I'm putting it into practice.

Once, I mentioned the obsessive thoughts to my psychiatrist, who wanted to give me Zyprexa, but I couldn't tolerate it. Why? I got dry mouth, dizzy and constipated, all common side effects. I read the side effects information and weight gain was one of them. The mind can be a powerful force. Since I've wrecked my bowel with laxatives, constipation in varying degrees is a constant companion, but I wonder if the dizziness and dry mouth were exaggerated by my fear of the weight gain side effects. Formerly, I would have rationalized away not taking the medication by honing in on the constipation. Although *anything* that produces even the slightest sluggishness in my bowels remains anathema to me, when ED had control, I would have used that crutch and never considered anything else. That's the kind of progress you make when you've lived with ED: one little step at a time.

I've found another way to deal with my obsessions. I now have an ongoing dialogue in my head. "Big deal, you ate a potato." I say to myself. Or, "Big deal, you're underwear doesn't match what you have on!" I find that talking to myself is therapeutic. People find me a bit odd if I forget and talk to myself out loud in the supermarket aisle, but, it works for me. Sometimes, I even ask God to kick the obsessive thoughts out of my mind. Sometimes, He does.

Reviewing the new tapes in my head is therapeutic for me, and allows me to say things to Art I simply couldn't in the past. Not the hurtful, cutting things I used to say, but ones that help us both to heal. When Art gets on my nerves, I say out loud, "It's your problem, not mine, and you're not going to get to me." It's become a signal between us that cuts through what once would have kicked off my repetitive cycle of repressed anger that ED loved so much. It helps Art realize that either he is pushing my buttons or my faulty wiring has misinterpreted what he said, allowing us to talk it out and avoid real problems.

As I slowly replace the old tapes, the tin cup bangs on the bars and the distant voice of ED from the dungeon wails, "Stop that, Pat. It's been important all your life. It's how you survive. You can't stop doing that now." So, I answer him. "Enough! Buzz off buster! I'm not listening to you any more."

Telling my story has also been therapeutic. It has allowed me to review the events of my past life with the knowledge I gained at Remuda, as well as to re-evaluate what went on at the Ranch and where I am now in relationship to then. I have not overcome, but am overcoming. I cannot believe that I allow ED to still occasionally threaten me, even after all the love and truth that I experienced at Remuda. I became sick and disgusted with myself when I realize how much I subconsciously try to cling to the lie that ruled my life for forty years.

After returning from Remuda, I continued my diary, and I'm glad I did. It's a living record of my recovery, and I will continue it as a means of daily review. It alerts me to the dangerous patterns that could lead to ED's escape from solitary confinement. As a secondary benefit, it gave me precise information about my progress since Remuda.

Of course, the thing I've had to change the most was my eating habits. Well it wasn't easy. I have developed the attitude that I have a terminal disease, and the only way I can keep on living is to take the medications that can stave off the grim reaper. The medication doesn't make you sick or cause your hair to fall out. Pasta, potatoes and rice lack those unpleasant side effects. As I obsess less, I live more.

When I lived in Ohio, I had no trouble going without food all day because I knew that I would eat dinner and leftovers then throw them back up. That's another treatment option I've adopted. I'm not euphemizing my disgusting behavior anymore. I didn't "lose it," I threw it up.

When I traveled back then, anorexia overwhelmed me. Hunger would consume me, and it took all my will to beat it down. After a time, I just didn't get hungry anymore. I suppose that is a blessing to those who are not purposely trying to starve themselves to death. To me, it was a sign of how much I was in control, and not of how out of control I truly was. Now, I eat on schedule, and that's no longer a problem.

I'm still trying to relearn what full and empty means. To totally succeed, I have to retrain my appetite center to behave in a normal fashion. I have to relearn that a tiny growl and that little empty feeling in the pit of my stomach is not the prelude to a panic attack that spawns abhorrent behavior. In fact, I actually get hungry now, and it doesn't drive me to a panic attack. I finally realize that food is not the enemy. I now have to embrace that realization as a way of life, but it's not easy.

When I first left Remuda, I ate sandwiches. I stopped because the numbers game in my head is so ingrained that I still haven't been able to totally erase it. When I realized that, the slip made me angry. Unlike the "bad old days," I didn't internalize the anger, convert it to gilt and trigger the ED cycle. I am determined to eat sandwiches again, and I'm getting there.

The same is true with frozen yogurt. Art and I would occasionally go out to TCBY for a treat. Art began to put on weight, which he did not welcome. He wanted to stop going out for yogurt, but gave me an alternative. He countered by buying TCBY yogurt bars so each of us could have one when we wanted it. That way, he wouldn't have to eat ice cream when I wanted it, particularly if he didn't want one at that time. It was a logical solution to my concerns.

I have always loved seeing Art and the rest of my family and friends, eat and enjoy foods, even those that I cannot force myself to eat. That's common for anorexics. What bad tape did I play to turn this situation into a problem? I was afraid I was starting to enjoy the ice cream too much. If there were ice cream bars at home, readily available, I could be tempted to eat them. If eating them made me feel too guilty, I would be in danger of the binge-barf cycle. The only solution I could see was to stop eating them, and discourage their presence in the house.

Then, from the dungeon, came ED's muffled whisper. "You know, Pat, it's much more convenient for Art to bring the ice cream in than to take the time to go out for ice cream with you. Why should he take the time? You're not worth it." Fortunately, I don't listen to the monster like I used to. My self esteem is better than that. And, Art doesn't have to prove anything to me. He's done that in spades.

I continue to fight falling back into my old ruts. Even though my eating is more normal now, I continue to eat the same breakfast and almost the same lunch every day. The foods are healthy, and many of them are things I wouldn't eat before. Still, I find security in their sameness. That's another thing on my to-do list. When we go out to eat, I nearly always gravitate to the "safe" foods on the menu. I know every salad in Las Vegas. Art is helping me with this, as he helps me with everything.

Although at the peak of my disease, I made a great show of wanting to go out for breakfast, or for lunch, I didn't enjoy eating. Most foods, when I looked at them on a plate at mealtime, made me physically ill unless they were safe foods such as lettuce with no dressing. Yet, when I did binge, I enjoyed the taste of what I was eating; until the guilt over my behavior became so overwhelming I had to purge. Thank God, most of that is gone, now. But, I admit, if I am in a restaurant and see grease dripping on the plate, I feel my stomach turn. I honestly don't think I'll ever be able to eat that kind of food again, but that's not such a bad thing.

However, I must be careful. Joanie gave me a list of "safe" desserts that are healthy, easy to prepare and that she thought I might enjoy. She encouraged me to try one of them. A friend who was visiting us encouraged me to try one. I used my new found independence and willingness to stand up for myself as a shield. I would do it when I was ready, and I wasn't ready. When I realized what I was doing, I decided to try again, and even went so far as to buy the ingredients. Somehow, I never found time to make it. I never said I was cured, but I'm working on it. Like Dirty Harry, "A gal's got to know her limitations." I know mine, and I'm working to change them.

Dinners at home are better than they used to be. I'm eating more foods, and I even got up enough gumption to use a little olive oil when I brown the beef for my Stroganoff, which I now eat *with* the noodles thank you. I still think about food, read cookbooks, and I love Emeril on the Food Channel. I haven't found the courage to try his recipes, because of the oil and butter he uses, but I have started adding a little oil to my fish before I grill them. Given time, God will work me though it all.

We love to hike and visit the national parks. On my last birthday, we were in Zion National Park, and we told the waiter in the restaurant it was my birthday. As a treat, he brought me two, chocolate dipped strawberries. I was able to eat one, but admit to feeling guilty about it. At least, I kept it down. Art relished the other one.

Thanks to my therapy, I have learned a great deal about my problem. Mealtime during my childhood was the chaos I have described. Though the meals were contentious, they were healthy and simple with a paucity of meat dishes. Mom was a decent cook, but with the ulcer-generating atmosphere of the table, I never learned to appreciate the food. My monster loved that and used it against me. Now, our table is a place of peace and tranquility, and I am enjoying it like never before.

In the old days, I customized my lifestyle to fit my disease perfectly. I have always been an early riser. I was up at the crack of dawn to get a running start on the day. My first task was to make myself a strong pot of coffee. The caffeine was necessary to jump start my nutritionally challenged system.

Now, my lifestyle has changed. Semi-retirement for me and retirement for Art has changed our lives to a leisurely, livable pace. I don't try to dodge anything, and I have completely changed to a healthier daily routine.

Mom never liked to cook, and it showed. I was determined to be better at it than she was. I don't have to prove anything to anybody now, except myself. I cook because I love cooking, and for no other reason.

I have also changed my food rituals. Most anorexics have them by the dozens.

The first is pushing the food around the palate. That's one that all of us with ED share. By using my fork to strategically rearrange things on my plate, it gave the impression I was eating when I wasn't. I didn't think anyone noticed it, but my family and friends all did.

The fork is a good weapon in the eating-not eating ritual. I would put a bite of food on my fork, make a gesture as though I was about to eat it, say something, and then put the fork down. Pick the fork up, ask a question, and put the fork down. Change the bite of food on the fork and start again. I fooled myself for years with that one.

Road to Recovery Potholes and All

Eating with the fingers ritual was my favorite. After ordering a salad, without dressing of course, I would pick up a single lettuce leaf and take a bite from it and replace it in the bowl. After a period of talking and gesturing, I would pick up another piece of lettuce, nibble a tiny bite from it, and replace it in the bowl. If there was bread handy, I liked to break off a piece of bread and keep it in my hand. Put it down for a moment, and then pick it up again. When I talked, I wanted to be sure everyone saw the bread in my hand. It proved I was eating, right? Wrong, it's merely a good show.

The tiny pieces ritual is another good one. Take one very small serving of meat. Cut off every millimeter of fat. Cut the remainder into pencil eraser size pieces or smaller, then chew and chew and chew. It also worked for vegetables. Starches were never a problem. I just didn't eat those.

Perhaps the most difficult thing to do was to look at a plate of food and see food. For the last forty years I have looked at a plate and seen a monster there, waiting to devour me. I shivered with fear every time I came near the dreaded beast. It was hard, but now I can sit down at the table without feeling nauseated with fear, and I can look at my stroganoff and see stroganoff. It's wonderful.

Bulimic behavior was almost too easy for me. I simply ate until I was so full I felt I was going to explode. Next, I bent over the commode, tightened my abdominal muscles like I was going to do a push up, then press my throat at the little notched area at the top of the breast bone. Bingo! Up came the hateful food.

More importantly, the binges were in response to intense hunger. My body was in a perpetual state of starvation. When I was exposed to even the slightest stress, that hunger came to the fore and I was as ravenous as a wolf after a hunting dry spell. When I gave into that hunger, it was a loss of control. By the time I had stuffed myself, the guilt over losing control set in. To ease the guilt, I threw up the food that caused the loss of control. It made me feel better.

Discovering the Monster Within

I learned an important lesson in that regard within the past few months. My older sister, Beverly, developed cancer of the esophagus and died after a long terrible bout with the disease. At her funeral, I became aware of that same intense hunger, and the urge to binge was nearly overwhelming. "Give in to it! Give into it and you'll feel better!" screamed ED's distant voice in my ear.

Although it was difficult, I didn't listen to him. Instead, I said, "Wait! I don't handle stress that way anymore. I'm sad for the loss of my sister and my friend. Giving in to aberrant behavior may make me feel better for the moment, but when it is over, those I loved will still be gone, and I'd have to do it again and again until time eased the pain of my loss. Instead, I will grieve for my loss, shed my tears and let it go.

When I arrived home in Las Vegas, a dear friend across the street died as well. The same feelings surfaced, but I recognized them at once for what they were. Now that I can do that, I won't let those feelings trap me again.

That part of binging is under control, but the foods that were the favorite fuel for my eating rampages still present problems for me. As a professional binger, I found there were foods that came up easily, like mashed potatoes, pasta, and ice cream. Others, like pizza, French fries, rice, and corn were hard to vomit up. I avoided them. Interestingly, my binge foods were also the comfort foods of my youth. I don't believe that was accidental.

I have been able to eat pasta and noodles again. Baked potatoes, or sweet potatoes I can handle, but I still have problems with the mashed variety. I've been able to do frozen yogurt, but real ice cream is not in my dietary scheme just yet. I'm working on all of them.

After years of hiding my emotions, it's hard to let them out in a normal channel, but I'm getting better at that, too. My friend and I had a disagreement as to which cast member of the original stable of zanies on "Saturday Night Live," had died of cancer. I was certain it was a person my friend was sure was alive. The person he said was dead I was positive was alive. The old Pat would have let it go. The new Pat stuck to her guns, and after a brisk back and forth exchange, a contemplative silence ensued. Suddenly, my friend came up with the correct name, and we both realized it at once.

Laughing, my friend complemented me on our debate. "That's really great, Pat," he said.

"Your willingness to take a stand and defend it like that tells me that you're cure is really going to stick."

And, I think he's right. With the improvement in my communications skills, on both the input and the output sides, replacing the bad tapes in my head with new ones, and my ability to spot the causes of my anxiety and deal with them makes me more than an even match for ED.

Although life remains a struggle in some areas, I cannot emphasize strongly enough the good things that have come from my battle with the monster. I now eat moderate amounts of food at each meal as well as a snack before bedtime. I eat pasta, potatoes baked or boiled, beef, pork, chicken, fish and shrimp. Cheese on salads, light sour cream in sauces and a little cooking oil spruce up what once was a very bland diet and makes me want to eat again. The occasional sandwich, tortilla chips and salsa, veggies beans chili and soup are back on my table. ED absolutely hates that!

Art and I like to explore the little, out-of-the-way towns in the west, and I no longer worry about a "good" restaurant being nearby. The new Pat's motto is, "a little unhealthy food won't kill us." That is such an amazing leap for me from my dysfunctional days of gain an ounce and die.

Using these new found skills, I've opened a dialog with my brother, and we are working on correcting a life time of misunderstandings. I have a better understanding of his situation, and hopefully he has a better understanding of mine. Dave was not dealt the best hand in life, but like his sister he's playing the cards the best that he can.

My sisters were able to talk with me about the abuses of our childhood, and it brought us closer together than ever before. Thank God we were able to do that before Beverly's death. God is at work in my life, and I realize that.

Perhaps the most exciting part of recovery is my new relationship with Art. Now, life is for us as it should have been for the last forty years. We are closer now than ever before. Our communications are honest and open. We're back to being best friends and buddies again. That doesn't mean we don't disagree and get bummed on occasion, but mending is easier and faster with open channels. We both need our space at times, but who doesn't. Neither of us have ever loved anyone else, and the fact that we are still together is a testimony to the man I married as well as that love. He is my friend, my confidant, my counselor, and he constantly watches my back lest I fall into old habits. My only regret is that I wasted so many years before I was able to get us back to this point in our relationship..

My health has improved, too. I told you I was a klutz, and that hasn't changed. Now my trips and falls are more likely to end in bruises and sprains rather than the skin tears and brakes of my ED days. I still have my team of angels with my from Internal Medicine, Urology, Psychiatry, Eye, Bone and Dietary specialties. I am very near my ideal weight for my size and health. At least that's what those who check the scale numbers tell me. I never look. Hopefully, I have my health problems under control and am repairing ED's major hits on my constitution. I don't want to call 911 anymore, especially since they put you on hold here in Las Vegas.

Why would I bother to tell my life story in such detail? The answer is understanding. The events in my life brought ED into it, and the rest of my life was affected by ED's presence. By telling my story, I hope to reach everyone from the teenager whose life if being consumed by being thin to the son, daughter, husband or wife of an anorexic all the way to the health professionals. My message is clear. I want to help people understand that the disease is *not about food*. It is about perception of self, life experiences and how one deals with them and the faulty tapes in their head.

Help is out there if we can recognize the symptoms and get help. Recognize the baggy clothing to hide the skeleton; force feeding others; bazaar eating habits like push the lettuce around the bowl, ice chewing, excessive chatter and jack-in-the-box behavior. "Self-help" has limited success, and self-denial remains the major stumbling blocks to cure. The disease is *curable*, even after years of affliction I know. I've been there; done that; got the T-shirt.

And, because I have been there, I think I can help others. I have already started by talking with a number of persons who either are personally struggling with the monster or who have a loved one who is. Working with my dietician, Joanie, we are setting up an eating disorder group therapy program coupled with a web site on eating disorders. It is not hard to recognize the tell-tale symptoms of anorexia, but is hard to get the person with the problem to admit that he or she needs help. Unless and until that happens, the monster will rule. I hope through education and personal experience to help others see what it took me four decades to see.

No, I don't plan to go into counseling. I have no professional training for that. I do plan to be an example; to share my life and my experiences; and to be a merchant of hope. Hope in an arena where it is a precious commodity.

Another positive is our new relationship with God. Both Art and I are regulars at the services and are part of a dynamic Bible study group. God is foremost in my heart and mind every single day. Art, too, has found the peace that passes all understanding. Life is good with God.

Of course, God is the biggest reason I am alive to tell my story. While I was trying to starve myself to death, He didn't send me any catastrophic illness to deal with. He didn't let me become involved in an auto accident or other trauma my body would not have been able to handle. And, He held my stomach together long enough for me to get enough nutrition on board so that I could survive the perforation and the surgery. If that wasn't enough, on our fortieth wedding anniversary, Art and I joined the Shadow Hills Church together.

Discovering the Monster Within

The realization that God loves me has done more to restore my self-esteem than anything else. God sees me as acceptable. He accepts me as I am, with all my faults and blemishes, and I don't have to change a thing about myself for Him to continue to love me. I'm valuable to him. Jesus himself said in Luke's Gospel, 12:24, "Look at the ravens. They don't need to plant or harvest or put food in barns because God feeds them. And you are far more valuable to him than any birds!" He thinks I'm loveable, because He sent His only son to save me. How awesome is that. And, He has forgiven me for the damage I have done to His temple, and believes I am capable of taking care of it now. With those kinds of confidences from The Big Guy, I very simply cannot fail.

I cannot fail; because I believe that God has given me the insight into my disease that one-day may allow me to help others with the same monster inside them. Art and I are playing a significant role in the life of Sarah, the wonderful young woman for whom we acted as surrogate parents at Remuda. We have continued parental-like support for her, and she is now a healthy, happy college student, who is well on her way to recovery. I hope to be able to help other young women realize the potential of who they are and what they can be.

Despite the trials in my life, I am a fortunate woman. I found my empty spot. All of us with ED have one. My empty spot was a lost childhood. Unwanted and abused, the chasm widened as my self esteemed bottomed out, and I became a poor imitation of other people's emotions. Then, I discovered I was a child of God with a family and friends who loved me. If I would let them, they would fill that void in my life, and smooth over the scars so I could live my life as a child of God rather than a victim of the monster.

In a box at the bottom of that empty spot in my life is the remnant of the little girl I put on hold when I abandoned her in my effort to survive. With God's help, I'm going to open that box and release the child that's inside. When I do my cure will be complete.

If I'm going to walk on water, I gotta get out of the boat. Well, I'm out of the boat! I'm out, and like the Apostle, Peter, I have my eyes on

Jesus. I know that I'm only a few steps away from the boat, but on my long and winding road I learned a lesson from Peter. I'll never take my eyes off the Master . . . ever!

The Beginning.

To order additional copies of

DISCOVERING THE
MONSTER
WITHIN

Have your credit card ready and call:

1-877-421-READ (7323)

or please visit our web site at
www.pleasantword.com

Also available at:
www.amazon.com
and
www.barnesandnoble.com

Printed in the United States
68580LVS00003B/278

9 781414 105994